Disease Eradication in the 21st Century

Implications for Global Health

Strüngmann Forum Reports

Julia Lupp, series editor

The Ernst Strüngmann Forum is made possible through the generous support of the Ernst Strüngmann Foundation, inaugurated by Dr. Andreas and Dr. Thomas Strüngmann.

This Forum was supported by funds from the Deutsche Forschungsgemeinschaft (German Science Foundation)

Disease Eradication in the 21st Century

Implications for Global Health

Edited by

Stephen L. Cochi and Walter R. Dowdle

Program Advisory Committee:
R. Bruce Alyward, Stephen L. Cochi, John O. Gyapong,
David Molyneux, Eric A. Ottesen, and Regina Rabinovich

The MIT Press

Cambridge, Massachusetts
London, England

© 2011 Massachusetts Institute of Technology and
the Frankfurt Institute for Advanced Studies

Series Editor: J. Lupp
Assistant Editor: M. Turner
Photographs: U. Dettmar
Design and realization: BerlinScienceWorks

MIT Press books may be purchased at special quantity discounts
for business or sales promotional use. For information, please email
special_sales@mitpress.mit.edu or write to Special Sales Department,
The MIT Press, 55 Hayward Street, Cambridge, MA 02142.

The book was set in TimesNewRoman and Arial.
Printed and bound in the United States of America.

Library of Congress Cataloging-in-Publication Data

Disease eradication in the 21st century : implications for global health /
edited by Stephen L. Cochi and Walter R. Dowdle.
    p. ; cm. — (Strüngmann Forum reports)
Includes bibliographical references and index.
ISBN 978-0-262-01673-5 (hardcover : alk. paper)
1. Communicable diseases—Prevention. 2. World health. I. Cochi, Stephen
L. II. Dowdle, Walter R. III. Series: Strüngmann Forum reports.
[DNLM: 1. Communicable Disease Control. 2. Immunization
Programs. 3. Socioeconomic Factors. 4. World Health.   WA 110]
RA643.D575   2011
362.196'9—dc23
                                                                2011014567

10 9 8 7 6 5 4 3 2 1

Contents

Governance

Disease Eradication and Health Systems

The Ernst Strüngmann Forum

Founded on the tenets of scientific independence and the inquisitive nature of the human mind, the Ernst Strüngmann Forum is dedicated to the continual expansion of knowledge. Through its innovative communication process, the Ernst Strüngmann Forum provides a creative environment within which experts scrutinize high-priority issues from multiple vantage points.

This process begins with the identification of themes. By nature, a theme constitutes a problem area that transcends classic disciplinary boundaries. It is of high-priority interest, requiring concentrated, multidisciplinary input to address the issues involved. Proposals are received from leading scientists active in their field and are selected by an independent Scientific Advisory Board. Once approved, a steering committee is convened to refine the scientific parameters of the proposal and select the participants. Approximately one year later, the central meeting, or Forum, is held to which circa forty experts are invited.

Preliminary discussion for this theme began shortly after I left the Dahlem Workshops to begin the process of establishing the program for the newly created Ernst Strüngmann Forum. Having worked previously with Walt Dowdle, Don Hopkins, Steve Cochi, and others on the 1997 Dahlem project, and in view of the changes that had taken place in global health initiatives since Dahlem, I was keen to learn whether the Forum could be of service to this sector again. Our talks expanded to include Eric Ottesen and Alan Hinman, and in September 2009, the steering committee—comprised of Bruce Aylward, Steve Cochi, Johnny Gyapong, David Molyneux, Eric Ottesen, and Regina Rabinovich—met to identify the key issues for debate and select the participants for the Forum, which was held in Frankfurt am Main, Germany, from August 29–September 3, 2010.

The activities and discourse surrounding a Forum begin well before participants arrive in Frankfurt and conclude with the publication of this volume. Throughout each stage, focused dialog is the means by which participants examine the issues anew. Often, this requires relinquishing long-established ideas and overcoming disciplinary idiosyncrasies that might otherwise inhibit joint examination. However, when this is accomplished, a unique synergism results and new insights emerge.

This volume conveys the synergy that arose from a group of diverse experts, each of whom assumed an active role, and is comprised of two types of contributions. The first provides background information on key aspects of the overall theme. These chapters have been extensively reviewed and revised to provide current understanding of the topics. The second (Chapters 7, 10, 14, and 19) summarizes the extensive group discussions that transpired. These chapters should not be viewed as consensus documents nor are they proceedings; they are intended to transfer the essence of the discussions, expose the open questions that still remain, and highlight areas in need of future enquiry.

In one area of the Forum—the group charged with discussing the critical components of the investment case for eradication and/or elimination initiatives (Chapter 10)—we soon realized that further work would be needed if a template for the investment case was to be created. Not wishing to lose momentum, a follow-up meeting for the group was proposed and additional expertise was brought in to complete the task. Hosted by Kim Thompson and Kid Risk, Inc. in Boston, this working session took place on December 9–10, 2010.

An endeavor of this kind creates its own unique group dynamics and puts demands on everyone who participates. Each invitee contributed not only their time and congenial personality, but a willingness to probe beyond that which is evident, and I wish to extend my gratitude to all. A special word of thanks goes to the steering committee, the authors of the background papers, the reviewers of the papers, and the moderators of the individual working groups: Regina Rabinovich, Chris Maher, Eric Ottesen, and Johnny Gyapong. To draft a report during the Forum and bring it to its final form in the months thereafter is no simple matter, and for their efforts, I am especially grateful to the rapporteurs: Kim Thompson, Kari Stoever, Peter Strebel, and Muhammad Ali Pate. Most importantly, I wish to extend my sincere appreciation to Steve Cochi and Walt Dowdle; their steady guidance throughout this project was invaluable and distinguished by their exemplary commitment.

A communication process of this nature relies on institutional stability and an environment that encourages free thought. The generous support of the Ernst Strüngmann Foundation, established by Dr. Andreas and Dr. Thomas Strüngmann in honor of their father, enables the Ernst Strüngmann Forum to conduct its work in the service of science. In addition, the following valuable partnerships are gratefully acknowledged: the Scientific Advisory Board, which ensures the scientific independence of the Forum; the German Science Foundation, which provided financial support for this theme; the Bill and Melinda Gates Foundation, whose support enabled the Boston meeting to be convened; and the Frankfurt Institute for Advanced Studies, which shares its vibrant intellectual setting with the Forum.

Long-held views are never easy to put aside. Yet, when this is achieved, when the edges of the unknown begin to appear and gaps in knowledge are able to be defined, the act of formulating strategies to fill these becomes a most invigorating exercise. It is our hope that this volume will convey a sense of this lively exercise and play its part in meeting the challenges of the global health landscape in the 21st century.

Julia Lupp, Program Director
Ernst Strüngmann Forum
http://www.esforum.de

List of Contributors

Jon Kim Andrus   Pan American Health Organization, Washington, D.C., U.S.A.

R. Bruce Aylward[*]   Global Polio Eradication Initiative, World Health Organization, 1211 Geneva 27, Switzerland

Dina Balabanova   Department of Global Health and Development, London School of Hygiene and Tropical Medicine, London WC1H 9SH, U.K.

Jeffrey Bates   UNICEF, New York, NY, U.S.A.

Robin Biellik   Consultant Epidemiologist, Geneva, Switzerland

Carlos Castillo-Solórzano   Pan American Health Organization, Washington, D.C., U.S.A.

Stephen L. Cochi   Global Immunization Division, Centers for Disease Control and Prevention, Atlanta, GA 30333, U.S.A.

Lesong Conteh   Institute for Global Health, Imperial College London, South Kensington Campus, London SW7 1NA, U.K.

Alya Dabbagh[*]   World Health Organization, 1211 Geneva 27, Switzerland

Ciro A. de Quadros   Sabin Vaccine Institute, Washington, D.C. 20006, U.S.A.

Lieven Desomer   UNICEF, New Delhi, India

Walter R. Dowdle   Task Force for Global Health, Decatur, GA 30030, U.S.A.

Radboud J. Duintjer Tebbens   Kid Risk, Inc., Newton, MA 02459, U.S.A.

Claudia I. Emerson   McLaughlin-Rotman Centre for Global Health, University of Toronto, Toronto, Ontario, M5G 1L7, Canada

Ulla Kou Griffiths   Department of Global Health and Development, London School of Hygiene and Tropical Medicine, London WC1H 9SH, U.K.

Sherine Guirguis   Communication for Development Specialist, Polio, UNICEF – India Country Office, New Delhi 110 003, India

John O. Gyapong   Ghana Health Service, Research and Development Division, Accra, Ghana

B. Fenton Hall   Division of Microbiology and Infectious Diseases, NIAID, NIH, DHHS, Bethesda, MD 20892-6604, U.S.A.

Robert G. Hall   Department of Epidemiology and Preventive Medicine, School of Public Health and Preventive Medicine, Monash University, Melbourne, Vic 3004, Australia

Piya Hanvoravongchai   Department of Global Health and Development, London School of Hygiene and Tropical Medicine, Faculty of Tropical Medicine, Bangkok 10400, Thailand

Donald A. Henderson   University of Pittsburg Medical Center, University of Pittsburg, Baltimore, MD, USA.

Alan R. Hinman   Task Force for Global Health, Decatur, GA 30030, U.S.A.

Adrian Hopkins   Task Force for Global Health, Decatur, GA 30030, U.S.A.

Dairiku Hozumi   PATH, Seattle, WA 98121, U.S.A.

Julie Jacobson   Bill & Melinda Gates Foundation, Seattle, WA 98102, U.S.A.

Ali Jaffer Mohamed   Ministry of Health, PC 113 Muscat, Sultanate of Oman

T. Jacob John   Kamalakshipuram, Vellore, TN 632002, India

Yayehyirad Kitaw   Private Consultant, Addis Ababa, Ethiopia

Tracey Koehlmoos   Health Systems and Infectious Diseases Division, International Center for Diarrhoeal Disease Research, Dhaka-1212, Bangladesh

Sebastião Loureiro   Instituto de Saude Coletiva, Federal University of Bahia, Salvador, Brazil

Chris Maher[*]   World Health Organization, 1211 Geneva 27, Switzerland

Mwelecele Malecela   Research Coordination and Promotion, National Institute for Medical Research, Daressalaam, Tanzania

Mitike Molla   School of Public Health, Addis Ababa University, Addis Ababa, Ethiopia

Thomas Moran[*]   WHO Headquarters, Polio Eradication, 1211 Geneva 27, Switzerland

Sandra Mounier-Jack   Department of Global Health and Development, London School of Hygiene and Tropical Medicine, London WC1H 9SH, U.K.

Linda Muller[*]   Global Polio Eradication Initiative, World Health Organization, 1211 Geneva 27, Switzerland

Jai Prakash Narain[*]   Communicable Diseases, WHO Regional Office for the South-East Asia Region, World Health House, New Delhi 11002, India

Ha Trong Nguyen   Hanoi School of Public Health, Hanoi, Vietnam

Valeria Oliveira Cruz   Department of Global Health and Development, London School of Hygiene and Tropical Medicine, London WC1H 9SH, U.K.

Pierre Ongolo-Zogo   Centre for Development of Best Practices in Health, Yaoundé Central Hospital, Yaounde, Cameroon

Eric A. Ottesen   Filariasis Support Center, Task Force for Global Health, 3 Decatur, GA 30030, U.S.A.

Muhammad Ali Pate   National Primary Health Care Development Agency, Garki, Abuja, Nigeria

Mirta Roses Periago   Pan American Health Organization, Washington, D.C., U.S.A.

Regina Rabinovich   Global Health Program, Bill & Melinda Gates Foundation, Seattle, WA 98102, U.S.A.

Umeda Sadykova   Dushanbe, Tajikistan

Harbandhu Sarma   Health Systems and Infectious Diseases Division, International Center for Diarrhoeal Disease Research, Bangladesh, Dhaka-1212, Bangladesh

Robert S. Scott   Rotary Foundation, International Polio Plus Committee, Cobourg, Ontario K9A 1N4, Canada

Peter A. Singer   McLaughlin-Rotman Centre for Global Health, Toronto, Ontario, M5G 1L7, Canada

Kari Stoever   GAIN – Global Alliance for Improved Nutrition, Washington, D.C. 20036, U.S.A.

Peter Strebel[*]   Immunization, Vaccines and Biologicals, World Health Organization, 1211 Geneva 27, Switzerland

Maria Gloria Teixeira   Instituto de Saude Coletiva, Federal University of Bahia, Salvador, Brazil

Kimberly M. Thompson   Kid Risk, Inc., Newton, MA 02459, U.S.A.

Nana A. Y. Twum-Danso   Project Fives Alive! Institute for Healthcare Improvement, c/o National Catholic Secretariat, Department of Health, Accra, Ghana

Stewart Tyson   Liverpool Associates in Tropical Health, Anson House, Liverpool, L3 5NY, U.K.

Jasim Uddin   Health Systems and Infectious Diseases Division, International Center for Diarrhoeal Disease Research, Bangladesh, Dhaka-1212, Bangladesh

Maya Vijayaraghavan   Global Immunization Division, Centers for Disease Control and Prevention, Atlanta, GA 30333, U.S.A.

Damian G. Walker Global Health Program, Bill & Melinda Gates Foundation, Seattle, WA 98102, U.S.A.

Ole Wichmann Immunization Unit, Robert Koch Institute, 13086 Berlin, Germany

Andy Wright Global Community Partnerships, GlaxoSmithKline, Brentford, Middlesex TW8 9GS, U.K.

---

* The views expressed in this publication reflect the individual perspectives of the participants and do not necessarily reflect the decisions, policy, or views of the World Health Organization.

1

The Eradication of Infectious Diseases

Understanding the Lessons and Advancing Experience

Stephen L. Cochi and Walter R. Dowdle

Introduction

Humankind has always been fascinated by scourges of disease that cause incalculable misery in the world and have a devastating impact on society, and by subsequent attempts to eradicate such diseases (D. R. Hopkins 2009). The sustained eradication of an infectious disease agent, in which humans are the primary or sole host, was achieved for the first (and only) time in 1980, when the World Health Assembly declared the world free of smallpox, following a campaign that began in 1959 and lasted nearly twenty years. Success in eradicating smallpox worldwide led to an increasingly intensive examination of the concepts and definitions associated with disease eradication, and the development of general and specific criteria as predictors of success for particular candidate diseases. The *Carter Center International Task Force for Disease Eradication* initiated a formal review of candidate diseases in 1988 and is currently completing a second review. The criteria for eradication were comprehensively examined at a workshop in 1997 on "The Eradication of Infectious Diseases" (Dowdle and Hopkins 1998), followed in 1998 by an expanded global forum on "Disease Eradication and Elimination as Public Health Strategies" (WHO 1998; CDC 1999a).

More than a decade has passed since the basic concepts and issues of eradication were systematically addressed. Meanwhile, considerable experience has been gained through the initiatives to eradicate polio and dracunculiasis (guinea worm), as well as in efforts to eliminate such diseases as measles, maternal and neonatal tetanus, onchocerciasis (river blindness), and lymphatic filariasis. Concepts of disease eradication have continued to evolve, influenced by scientific advances, field experiences, societal and ethical issues, and economic realities.

The need to convene this forum was especially timely since heightened interest in the potential eradication of various infectious diseases is once again moving front and center. For example, at the May 2008 meeting of the Executive Board of the World Health Assembly, the Board requested that WHO examine the feasibility of global measles eradication and report back to the Board in 2010. Also in 2008, both the WHO and the Bill & Melinda Gates Foundation publicly called for development of a program of work to achieve malaria eradication in the longer term (30+ years). These examples are illustrative of the ongoing fascination with the concept of eradication. However, they also demonstrate the continuing need to ensure that such initiatives are carefully considered, based on a full understanding of the biological, political, social, and economic complexities associated with a successful eradication program. With increasing interest in identifying candidate diseases for eradication, these complexities need to be addressed for the benefit of public health decision makers, politicians, scientists, and the world at large. In addition, the rapid accumulation of knowledge since the 1990s and the radical changes in the global landscape necessitate an in-depth, systematic reassessment and reexamination of eradication in the context of global health in the 21st century.

The central meeting of this *Ernst Strüngmann Forum* on "Disease Eradication in the Context of Global Health in the 21st Century" took place in Frankfurt, Germany, from August 29 to September 3, 2010. It brought together a diverse group of experts from academia, government and research agencies, international multilateral organizations, nongovernmental development organizations and foundations, the pharmaceutical industry, and the private sector. Participants were drawn from around the globe as well as from the many different disciplines that impact global health, including infectious disease, epidemiology, public health and preventive medicine, health economics, health policy and management, health systems research, and medical ethics.

Those who attended were acutely mindful that they were carrying on the legacy of those before them who have studied and discussed the concepts of disease eradication and grappled with its complexities. As Thomas Jefferson, in the early 1800s, wrote to Edward Jenner, the developer of the first smallpox vaccine: "Yours is the comfortable reflection that mankind can never forget that you have lived. Future nations will know by history only that the loathsome smallpox has existed."

This Forum, through a combination of plenary discussions and focused small group deliberations on specific critical issues, conducted an in-depth, systematic reassessment and reexamination of eradication in the context of global health in the 21st century. The goals of this Forum were determined as follows:

- to assess the applicability, in the present and near-term future, of infectious disease eradication and elimination as components of the global health landscape;
- to explore the prospects, feasibility, and challenges of disease eradication/elimination initiatives; and
- to develop a framework for a priority-setting process to enable the identification of the most appropriate targets for disease eradication as well as the critical factors for success.

Lessons from previous and current eradication programs were examined, and the collective experience and knowledge of the Forum participants were used to extend global consensus on a variety of challenging issues. Each of four work groups focused on a specific set of issues as the central focus of their group discussions and reported back to the entire group. The scheduling permitted substantial opportunities for cross-fertilization through the participation and exchange of ideas across groups, an exchange that continued well after the final session in Frankfurt. Building on the progress achieved in Frankfurt, a follow-up meeting was convened in Boston from December 9–10, 2010, to expand the discussion on the critical components of the investment case for eradication and/or elimination initiatives.

Evolution of Current Concepts and Definitions

The terms disease *eradication* and disease *elimination* describe ideal outcomes of disease control, where *control* is defined as the reduction of disease morbidity/mortality to a locally acceptable level (Fenner et al. 1998; Hinman 1984). The 1997 Dahlem Workshop attempted to better define the two terms by using current models and building on earlier definitions (Ottesen et al. 1998). Elimination was defined in two categories according to whether the indigenous agent remained (e.g., *Clostridium tetani*) or no longer remained (e.g., wild poliovirus) in the specific geographical area (Ottesen et al. 1998:48):

> Elimination of disease: Reduction to zero of the incidence of a specified disease in a defined geographic area as a result of deliberate efforts; continued intervention measures are required. [The model was neonatal tetanus.]

> Elimination of infection: Reduction to zero of the incidence of infection caused by a specific agent in a defined geographic area as a result of deliberate efforts; continued measures to prevent reestablishment of transmission are required. [The model was the 1994 declaration of the Americas as polio-free.]

The former was seen as the highest possible achievement for neonatal tetanus, the latter as a geographic step toward global polio eradication. The definition of eradication followed along the lines of common usage (Ottesen et al. 1998:48):

Permanent reduction to zero of the worldwide incidence of infection caused by
a specific agent as a result of deliberate efforts; intervention measures are no
longer needed. [The model was smallpox.]

This definition of eradication implied a state of global permanence and conveyed the programmatic and economic advantages of eradication.

Events Since Dahlem

In 1998, at the conference on "Global Disease Elimination and Eradication
as Public Health Strategies" (WHO 1998; CDC 1999a) in Atlanta, some participants objected to the use of the term elimination, arguing that the distinction between eradication and elimination was artificial, confusing, not directly
translatable in many languages, and not easily understood by people outside
of international public health inner circles. The post-conference ad hoc group
appointed to resolve the issue combined the two terms and defined eradication
as (CDC 1999a:152):

The absence of a disease agent in nature in a defined geographical area as a result
of deliberate control efforts. Control measures can be discontinued when the risk
of disease importation is no longer present.

De Serres et al. (2000) noted that the Dahlem definition of elimination as "reduction to zero" was unrealistic and functionally unnecessary. They proposed
to define elimination as a situation in which sustained transmission cannot occur and secondary spread from importation will end naturally.

In 2001, the anthrax attacks in the United States prompted some individuals to question publicly the concept of eradication, and the creation of opportunities for bioterrorism in increasingly nonimmune populations in a smallpox, polio, and possibly measles-free world. Since then, public concern over smallpox
virus as an agent of bioterrorism has gradually subsided. However, allaying national security concerns over the phrase "intervention measures are no longer
needed" is only possible for those parasitic diseases where agent eradication
and extinction are synonymous.

In 2002, the national security debate was further stimulated by the report
(Cello et al. 2002) that infectious poliovirus had been created in the laboratory
following a recipe downloaded from the internet and using gene sequences
from a mail-order supplier. Discontinuing intervention efforts, seen as justification for eradication in the smallpox model, became, in the views of some,
justification for discontinuing disease eradication efforts, which ignores the
"natural terrorism" of eradicable diseases that is the real threat to the world's
poorest populations on a daily basis.

However, if the geographical qualifiers are removed from the Dahlem definitions, as proposed by the Atlanta group in 1998, and if the intervention qualifiers are removed because of national security concerns, what remains of the

definition of eradication is: the absence of the disease agent in a defined geographical area as a result of deliberate control efforts.

This minimalist definition is not unlike that proposed by Andrews and Langmuir nearly fifty years ago as the "purposeful reduction of specific disease prevalence....to the point of continued absence of transmission within a specified area" (Andrews and Langmuir 1963:1). With this definition, elimination becomes redundant, national security becomes a non-issue, post-eradication intervention practices become optional according to the diseases and national policy, and eradication becomes national, regional, or global.

Definitions from This Forum

The minimalist definition was dismissed by Forum participants on the grounds that it conveyed too little information. After much discussion during and after the Forum, the following definitions emerged:

> *Global eradication*: The worldwide absence of a specific disease <u>agent</u> in nature as a result of deliberate control efforts that may be discontinued where the agent is judged no longer to present a significant risk from extrinsic sources (e.g., smallpox).

The major difference between this definition of eradication and the Dahlem version is that the proposed definition permits the post-eradication flexibility for national health authorities to consider on the basis of risk when control efforts may be discontinued.

> *Regional or national eradication*: The absence of a specific disease <u>agent</u> in a defined geographic area as a result of deliberate control efforts that must be continued to prevent reestablished endemic transmission (e.g., polio, measles, rubella, guinea worm).

The context here assumes that the "defined geographic area" is substantially large and populous to give credibility to the claim that sustained eradication has been achieved.

> *Elimination*: The absence of a <u>disease</u> caused by a specific agent in a defined geographic area as a result of deliberate control efforts that must be continued in perpetuity to prevent reemergence of disease (e.g., neonatal tetanus).

Most discussion at the Forum centered on use of the term elimination, particularly as a step toward global eradication. Some meeting participants expressed the opinion that the term elimination had been firmly implanted in the lexicon of the international health community, particularly in neglected tropical disease programs, and should therefore not be discarded. The measles group, for example, has stated on record that it prefers to reserve use of the term eradication exclusively for global achievements and the term elimination for subglobal (e.g., regional) geographic achievements (WHO 2010e). Other meeting participants challenged the focus on established human diseases, and suggested that the definitions might exclude important accomplishments related to stopping emerging diseases, including the successful disruption of transmission of severe acute respiratory syndrome (SARS).

The intent of this Forum is not to establish a consensus document or exclusive definitions, but to identify shortcomings of the Dahlem definitions and offer possible solutions. Definitions are, and will continue to be, established through broad acceptance and popular usage.

Criteria for Disease Eradication Programs

Biological and Technical Feasibility

Although our definition of disease agents for eradication and elimination clearly included biological and technical feasibility, we emphasize the importance of these in the context of disease eradication programs. There are distinct biological features of an organism as well as technical tools and tactics that determine the potential eradicability of an organism (Hinman and Hopkins 1998; Aylward et al. 2000a; Dowdle 1998; Keegan et al. 2011). The categorization of a disease as not eradicable or difficult to eradicate can change completely if research efforts are successful in developing new and effective intervention tools. This demonstrates the central and important role of research in any eradication program. For purposes of this volume, we identified four indicators of primary importance:

1. An effective, practical intervention must be available to interrupt transmission of the agent.
2. Practical diagnostic tools must exist with sufficient sensitivity and specificity to detect levels of infection that can lead to transmission.
3. There must be an absence of a nonhuman reservoir (when humans are essential for the life cycle of the agent), and the organism does not amplify in the environment.
4. Success of the eradication strategy must be demonstrated in a large geographic area or region.

Past failures of eradication programs have been largely attributable to failure of the interventions or strategies, providing a cautionary note of the need to understand the natural history and biology of the disease thoroughly as a fundamental precept when considering an eradication or elimination program. For example, nonhuman primates were found to harbor yellow fever virus in 1915, and malaria mosquito vectors eventually became resistant to the insecticides (Aylward et al. 2000a). In the case of yaws, the prevalence and importance of inapparent infections were underestimated.

Societal and Political Support

Despite strong biological, technical, and cost-benefit arguments for a particular eradication initiative, securing societal and political commitment is now recognized as a substantial challenge (Aylward et al. 2000b). An appreciation of societal and political considerations is critical in transforming eradication programs from technically feasible efforts into operationally successful initiatives (Hinman and Hopkins 1998; Aylward et al. 2000a; Dowdle 1998; Keegan et al. 2011; Aylward et al. 2000b; Henderson 1987; Cochi et al. 1998; Hall, this volume). The success of such initiatives is dependent on a consistently high level of political and societal commitment from the beginning to the end. Societal and political support in industrialized countries is also essential for mobilizing external resources for eradication in developing countries. Explicit efforts to identify countries with weak societal or political commitment must be central to evaluating the overall feasibility of any proposed eradication effort. Some of the key questions that arose during our discussions include:

- What organizational arrangements and institutional obligations are appropriate to disease eradication or elimination programs (see Stoever et al., this volume)?
- What are the most appropriate governance models (see Stoever, this volume)?
- What is the meaning of disease eradication or elimination to politicians, non-scientists, and others outside the health field (see Strebel et al., Bates et al., and Emerson, this volume)?
- What are the major political challenges in current eradication initiatives (see Hall, this volume)?
- What has been learned about political and community mobilization, and how do we build this into future eradication initiatives (see Bates et al., Pate et al., Hinman, Tyson and Biellik, Hanvoravongchai et al., all this volume)?

Economic Considerations

Economic evaluations of health interventions play an increasing role in resource allocation decisions (Hall, this volume; Barrett 2004; Thompson and Duintjer Tebbens 2007; Duintjer Tebbens et al. 2011; Thompson and Duintjer Tebbens, and Thompson et al., this volume). Decisions have to be made as to whether the use of finite resources for a disease eradication or elimination program is preferable to their use in nonhealth sector projects, other health interventions, or direct investments in the overall health system. Formal economic analytical methods are not ideally suited to eradication programs; one of the most significant challenges relates to valuing the direct and indirect benefits of elimination nationally and eradication globally (Thompson and Duintjer

Tebbens, this volume). It can be difficult for politicians and the public to recognize the value of prevention and the savings associated with not incurring disease or treatment costs that an eradication program offers. These are global public goods.

Among the questions addressed at the Forum were the following:

- What are the critical components of the investment case for eradication and/or elimination initiatives (see Thompson et al., Walker et al., this volume)?
- Is there common ground for evaluating proposed eradication initiatives on economic and humanitarian criteria (see Thompson and Duintjer Tebbens, Thompson et al., and Walker et al., this volume)?
- Can a consensus be reached on the complexity and uniqueness inherent in applying economic principles to eradication programs (Thompson et al. and Walker et al., this volume)?
- Can humanitarian benefits be quantified (Thompson and Duintjer Tebbens, this volume)?

Linkage with Health Systems and Delivery of Other Health Interventions

To be successful, eradication initiatives of the 21st century must balance the need for an obsessive, laser-like focus to achieve specific goals and objectives (D. R. Hopkins 2009) with a demonstration that such initiatives will positively interact with the broad-based, primary health care system (WHO Maximizing Positive Synergies Collaborative Group 2009; Melgaard et al. 1998; Atun et al. 2008; Taylor and Waldman 1998). Eradication and ongoing primary health care programs represent potentially complementary approaches to public health; areas of both synergy and tension exist that must be recognized and addressed. Efforts are needed to identify and characterize those factors that maximize positive interactions and minimize negative or harmful effects. Experience shows that negative effects are more likely to manifest themselves in countries where the health infrastructure is weak. A recent review encouraged "the creation of a new framework in which the disease-specific and health systems approaches are mutually interdependent and have a common goal to improve the health of all people" (WHO Maximizing Positive Synergies Collaborative Group 2009:2161). Questions that were addressed at the Forum included:

- What is the optimal use of resources for delivering additional health interventions in the context of disease eradication initiatives, and vice versa (Pate et al., Hinman, and Tyson and Biellik, this volume)?
- What are the mutual benefits of eradication initiatives and a functioning community health delivery system (Pate et al., Hinman, Tyson and Biellik, and Hanvoravongchai et al., this volume)?
- When do vertical (stand-alone) programs have a place in health systems (Hinman, this volume)?

Lessons from Previous and Current Eradication Programs

A number of excellent reviews draw broad lessons from previous eradication program experiences that we find quite instructive when considering whether to embark on a specific disease eradication initiative (Hinman and Hopkins 1998; Aylward et al. 2000b; Dowdle 1998; Keegan et al. 2011; Aylward et al. 2000a; Henderson 1987). Hinman and Hopkins (1998) provided a list of ten main lessons from these collective experiences:

1. Understand the natural history of the disease thoroughly.
2. Consult widely before embarking on eradication.
3. Initiate surveillance early and use surveillance information to guide program strategy.
4. Eradication programs require a vertical approach.
5. Remain open minded and flexible; expect the unexpected.
6. Some countries may need more help than others.
7. Coordination of external donors is essential.
8. Political commitments from all levels are essential.
9. Inspire enthusiasm, but don't declare success prematurely.
10. Set a specific target date for eradication.

These general lessons are enriched by insights gained from comparative analyses of the successes and failures of previous eradication programs (Aylward et al. 2000b; Dowdle 1998; Keegan et al. 2011). A fundamental lesson is that neither biological nor technical feasibility—although essential, critically necessary elements of success—are sufficient criteria to be fulfilled in isolation. Additional nonbiological factors are ultimately the key to successful eradication efforts. Such evaluations have focused on political, social, economic, health system, leadership and management, and other factors that must be weighed as evidence for or against the establishment of an eradication initiative (Aylward et al. 2000b; Dowdle 1998; Keegan et al. 2011; Aylward et al. 2000a; Henderson 1987; Hall, this volume).

The Way Forward

The issues addressed at this Forum illustrate how much has been learned and the wealth of experience gained over the past twenty years regarding the conception, formulation, planning, and implementation of various disease eradication and elimination programs. However, this Forum also illustrates the need for many more efforts to enlarge our knowledge base, experience, and understanding of this particular public health approach to conquering disease and human affliction. Eradication of disease is, in fact, the ultimate aspirational goal of public health; however, this powerful tool is potentially applicable to only a limited number of diseases in the current era. The history of past failed eradication initiatives teaches us the critical need to exercise rigor and apply the lessons from these experiences as we contemplate embarking on new eradication or elimination programs. When considering such programs, nothing short of a systematic, comprehensive analysis of feasibility is needed, including a full examination of the challenges and opportunities of a decision to move forward, and the factors associated with likelihood of success or failure. This Forum describes the careful and deliberate evaluations that are required. When attributes and potential benefits are favorable, the way forward becomes clear.

Lessons Learned from Current Elimination and Eradication Initiatives

2

Lessons from the Late Stages of the Global Polio Eradication Initiative

R. Bruce Aylward

Abstract

Given the substantial influence that the Global Polio Eradication Initiative can be expected to have on future eradication initiatives, it seems increasingly important to identify and analyze lessons from each phase of this program. The protracted "tail" of the polio eradication initiative currently appears to be disproportionately influencing discussion of, and decisions on, future eradication efforts, particularly with respect to the potential merits of a future measles eradication effort. Consequently, for the purposes of this chapter the "late stages" of the polio initiative have been analyzed, with most attention to those geographical areas that have never interrupted wild poliovirus transmission and those which have been regularly reinfected. The major lessons that have been identified might be applied earlier in future eradication initiatives, ultimately increasing the prospects for their launch, early scale-up, and successful conclusion. The most pertinent lessons identified were in assessing operational feasibility, sustaining and applying research, conducting effective advocacy at the subnational level, operating in insecure areas, and anticipating and addressing vulnerabilities in areas with especially weak health systems.

Introduction

Launched in 1988 through a resolution of the World Health Assembly, the Global Polio Eradication Initiative (GPEI) has grown to become one of the most ambitious, internationally coordinated health initiatives in history (Fine and Griffiths 2007), and certainly the largest eradication effort to date. At its peak of field operations, the program directly employed over 4000 people globally, managed an annual budget of approximately USD 1000 million, and maintained active field operations in more than 75 countries (WHO 2003a). Each year, millions of people were engaged to vaccinate hundreds of millions of children in multiple mass vaccination campaigns with oral poliovirus vaccine (OPV).

Consequently, the GPEI may offer insights to facilitate the pursuit of future eradication initiatives, particularly against widespread, highly contagious but vaccine-preventable pathogens such as the measles virus.

This article takes as its starting point the operational and technical challenges that the GPEI has faced since the year 2000, the original target date for interrupting wild poliovirus transmission globally (WHO 1988). Many of the lessons from the earlier launch and scale-up of the GPEI are either self-evident or documented elsewhere (Aylward et al. 2003; Aylward and Linkins 2005). Furthermore, lessons from the late stages of this initiative may have the greatest implications for improving the speed and efficiency of future eradication efforts, thereby avoiding the inevitable problems of fatigue and waning confidence associated with setbacks and missed milestones. This perspective also seemed most relevant to the international dialog on eradication at the end of 2010, as the GPEI's "late stage" challenges appeared to be having the greatest influence, whether consciously or unconsciously, on that debate and especially in the context of a future measles eradication effort.

Context

Although the GPEI was launched in 1988, most polio-infected countries initiated eradication activities only in the mid-1990s, with the last two countries (Democratic Republic of the Congo and Sierra Leone) only beginning in 2000 (Figure 2.1). A combination of global, regional, and country-specific factors was responsible for the delays. Available financing was part of the equation, but in some areas there was simply a lack of sociopolitical "buy-in" to the global eradication goal, ranging from that of key health authorities to the broader sociopolitical environment. This reflected the lack of commitment to the fundamental eradication strategies by many public health officials and an insufficient understanding and acceptance of the enormity of the operational challenges to implement them globally (WHO 2008b). Thus the successful adaptation and implementation of the original Pan American Health Organization (PAHO) polio eradication strategies in the Western Pacific Region of the World Health Organization (WHO) was pivotal, as it provided the proof of "operational" feasibility in large population countries (China) and fragile states (Cambodia in the early 1990s) that many decision makers seemed to require.

As polio eradication efforts scaled up rapidly in other areas of the world, progress was dramatic (Figure 2.1). In contrast to the misconception that most countries have been trying to eradicate polio for over twenty years, the average time from strategy initiation to interruption of indigenous wild poliovirus was only two to three years (Figure 2.2). The few areas that remained "endemic" by the mid-2000s were the exceptions. However, it is these "exceptional" areas of

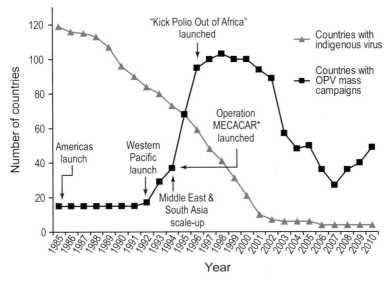

Figure 2.1 Countries with indigenous poliovirus circulation versus the initiation of national eradication efforts, 1985–2006.

northern Nigeria, northern India, southern Afghanistan, and Pakistan, as well as the nearby countries which regularly became reinfected, which may have the most relevant lessons for future eradication efforts.

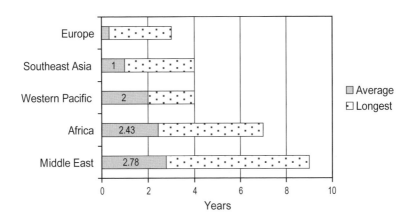

Figure 2.2 Time to interrupt indigenous wild poliovirus transmission after initiation of OPV mass campaigns, by WHO Region, excluding the Americas and currently "endemic" countries (Afghanistan, India, Nigeria, Pakistan).

Major Lessons Learned

The late stages of the GPEI offer five major lessons for consideration by future eradication initiatives.

Operational Feasibility: Establish Compelling Proof
from the Outset in a Range of Difficult Settings

Three criteria are usually cited in assessing the feasibility of eradicating a human pathogen (Dowdle and Hopkins 1998; Goodman et al. 1998a). First is "biologic" feasibility: humans must be essential to the life cycle of the pathogen, there should be no chronic-carrier state, and the eradication tools/strategy should have demonstrated efficacy in diagnosing infection and interrupting transmission on a large geographical scale. The second is the "cost-benefit" criterion: it should be possible to recoup the marginal costs of moving from control to eradication within a reasonable, finite time period (e.g., 20 years). Although least understood and measurable, the third set of criteria is "societal and political": this support should be sufficient to maintain an intensive, costly effort over the 10- to 20-year period that will probably be needed to achieve and certify eradication.

The late stages of the GPEI demonstrate that proof of technical feasibility in the Western Hemisphere (or in any single, largely homogenous area) does not necessarily equate to operational feasibility in all potential settings and conditions under which eradication strategies will need to be applied. On the contrary, while proof-of-principle in the Americas is certainly *necessary* before embarking on global eradication of a pathogen, it is probably no longer *sufficient* for marshalling the commitments needed to launch new eradication initiatives, as evidenced in part by the reticence, as of 2010, of major development agencies to embrace measles eradication (Obadairo 2010).

Evidence that a new eradication initiative meets an additional, explicit criterion of "operational feasibility" should enhance its prospects for both success and support. The specifics for concluding whether "operational feasibility" has been established will differ by pathogen. For widespread, highly contagious pathogens such as polio, the GPEI suggests operational feasibility might prove most convincing if achieved in areas with particularly weak health systems, fragile or failed states, high-population density areas, large federated republics and, ideally, places with a combination of these characteristics. For vaccine-preventable diseases, this can be visualized as the areas where the immunity threshold for interrupting transmission is highest and areas where the difference between the threshold and current population immunity levels is greatest (Figure 2.3).

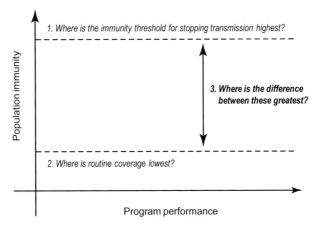

Figure 2.3   Schematic for identifying areas where demonstration of the *operational feasibility* of eradication may be most compelling.

Subnational Leaders: Establish Robust Mechanisms to Understand and Engage Them

Meeting the logistical challenges of OPV mass campaigns that cover an entire country in a very short period of time requires resources (e.g., human, transport, communications) far beyond those of the health sector. Consequently, the GPEI's advocacy efforts were initially focused on engaging national leaders, especially in countries with very weak health systems, to access complementary systems and ensure the accountability needed to reach most children during each OPV mass campaign.

While this strategy was largely successful, it was simply inadequate in large, federated republics, where subnational leaders controlled such resources (e.g., Nigeria, Pakistan, and India). Unfortunately, engaging directly with subnational leaders, beyond technical or operational issues, can be problematic for agencies whose official dealings are at the national level. However, such leaders may ultimately control the fate of a global eradication effort, as was demonstrated most famously by the prolonged suspension of polio vaccination in one state of northern Nigeria in 2003 (Kaufmann and Feldbaum 2009).

Recognizing this reality, future eradication initiatives would benefit greatly by establishing from the outset strategies, advocates, and processes to systematically access and engage subnational leaders in key countries. In the GPEI, this work was greatly facilitated by the decision of Rotary International, one of the four spearheading partners, to establish "National *PolioPlus* Committees" in most polio-infected countries. With 1.2 million members worldwide, often leading figures in their communities, Rotarians have played a central role in the GPEI's subnational advocacy, working in close collaboration with technical counterparts in WHO and UNICEF.

Research: Sustain an Intensive Program of
Work throughout the Initiative

Contrary to one of the more intractable myths about the GPEI, the initiative has, since its inception, pursued an active research agenda across a wide range of issues, though with varying intensity and focus depending on the challenges it faced or anticipated at any given time. Curiously, the GPEI often found itself having to defend such investments, as some enthusiasts argued that proof of principle had long been established and success was simply a matter of implementing standard strategies.

Such an attitude failed to appreciate the case for ongoing research, part of which can be illustrated with GPEI examples. First, it is simply not possible to anticipate the obstacles that may be encountered when applying strategies developed in one geographic area of the world to global contexts and cultures. Research is needed to optimize application (e.g., the problem of lower OPV efficacy in northern India) (Grassly et al. 2006). Second, given that an eradication initiative can take decades to complete, an active research agenda is key to ensuring major developments are exploited in areas such as diagnostics, vaccinology, and cold-chain technology to enhance program effectiveness and reduce cost (e.g., vaccine vial monitors, real-time PCR). Third, an active research agenda allows an eradication program to investigate and adapt to aspects of the pathogen or its control that were unrecognized at the outset (e.g., circulating vaccine-derived polioviruses) (Kew et al. 2005).

The GPEI's capacity to maintain an active research program was greatly facilitated by the U.S. Centers for Disease Control and Prevention (CDC), another of the four spearheading partners, which brought its epidemiologic and virological expertise to the program. Grants from the Bill & Melinda Gates Foundation (BMGF) and the Global Alliance for Vaccines and Immunization (GAVI) both played important roles in financing major research projects, particularly in the areas of new vaccine development and testing (El-Sayed et al. 2008; Sutter et al. 2010). Perhaps most important was establishing a dedicated research and product development team within the Polio Eradication Initiative at WHO headquarters in Geneva. This team was fundamental to the successful coordination of the network of vaccine manufacturers, academic research institutions, not-for-profit research groups, public health laboratories, and regulatory agencies worldwide that facilitated the often fast-track development, testing and licensing of new vaccines, diagnostics and related technologies, as well as operations research. That said, a key research area that has yet to be optimized is the area of social science research: future initiatives should also recognize from the outset the need for strong capacity to rapidly conduct or commission such work.

Insecurity and Conflict: Ensure Program Capacity to Study and Adapt in Each Setting

The GPEI is often cited for its success in implementing strategies in conflict-affected areas (Hull 2007; Bush 2000). In fact, this experience is frequently held up as evidence that "polio can be eradicated anywhere," with the allure of tactics such as "Days of Tranquillity" capturing the imagination of supporters. While this may be broadly true, such statements fail to capture the complexity of conflict and the constant need to adapt tactics to operate with at least some degree of safety in such settings. For example, the conflict-related challenges the GPEI faces in southern Afghanistan and the Federally Administered Tribal Areas of Pakistan in the late stages of the global initiative are substantively different from those it had to address earlier in areas such as Somalia and the Democratic Republic of the Congo (Tangermann et al. 2000).

In reality, success in eradicating polio from one conflict-affected or insecure area did not "prove" the overall feasibility of the global task; it did, however, provide invaluable experience that could be brought to the next such challenge. Common principles exist, particularly that people living in conflict-affected areas are highly motivated to improve their children's futures and can be readily engaged in the delivery of basic health services. Similarly, major humanitarian actors (e.g., the International Committee of the Red Cross) can provide invaluable assistance in negotiating access and vetting potential local collaborators. Working from such fundamentals, a range of tactics were developed and employed to access children and boost immunity more rapidly in these areas, including Days of Tranquillity, "access negotiators," and OPV "Short Interval Additional Dose" campaigns to exploit brief windows of opportunity. Just as important were the more mundane lessons learned on how to establish and sustain administrative processes to contract services and move resources in such settings.

Recognizing that insecurity and conflict will be a continuing challenge in the future, new eradication initiatives should from the outset:

- Recruit individuals with expertise in conflict, political mapping, and associated skills.
- Build the capacity to support teams and workers in conflict-affected areas.
- Identify and engage nontraditional partners and decision makers.
- Refine tactics and technologies to simplify work in such settings (e.g., hand-held jet injectors for administering vaccines).

As of the end of 2010, there is no evidence that, with the appropriate investments and attention, conflict should pose an insurmountable barrier to achieving an eradication goal.

Weak Health Systems: Sustain Gains by Addressing System Vulnerabilities

The stalling of polio eradication progress during the period 2004–2008 in the last four "endemic" countries soon led to a second major problem for the GPEI: the recurrent reinfection of previously polio-free areas (Figure 2.4) (WHO 2010f). Although OPV mass campaigns could rapidly interrupt indigenous poliovirus in areas with very weak health systems, campaigns were less effective in preventing new outbreaks following virus importations. Multiple factors contributed to this problem, especially the drop in OPV campaign quality that was often observed once transmission had been interrupted. In addition, the impact of the original campaigns in these settings may have been augmented by the contribution that circulating indigenous viruses had made to population immunity.

Consequently, countries with a combination of weak health systems and strong trade, cultural, and other links with polio endemic areas suffered a disproportionate number of polio importations and outbreaks, particularly in West and Central Africa and the Horn of Africa (WHO 2010f; O'Reilly et al., submitted). The subsequent human and financial costs were enormous, with thousands of children paralyzed and hundreds of millions of dollars expended in outbreak response activities. Clearly, the most important lesson from this experience is the importance of coordinating global eradication efforts to minimize the risk of reinfecting pathogen-free areas. However, as there will always be delays in some countries, it is essential to (a) plan and budget for sustained, intensive activities (e.g., OPV campaigns) in areas with a combination of weak

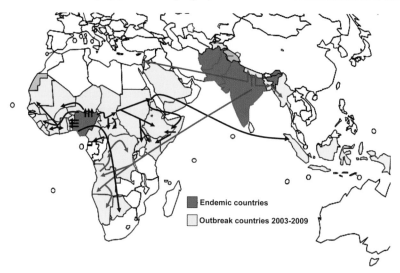

Endemic countries

Outbreak countries 2003-2009

Figure 2.4 International spread of wild polioviruses into previously polio-free areas, 2003–2009.

health systems and a high risk of reinfection due to strong links with an endemic area (O'Reilly et al., submitted), and (b) establish from the outset specific plans, responsibilities, and accountabilities for strengthening the underlying health systems, starting with highest risk countries and areas.

Recognizing that health systems strengthening is generally a long-term agenda of work, eradication programs need to map and engage *all* of the local systems (e.g., education, defense, transport, information) that can be exploited to access populations in countries with particularly weak health systems and a high risk of reinfection. This sometimes requires an attitude shift to appreciate the invaluable complementary role of such systems, and to refocus the health system on the mobilization and management of those complementary systems to facilitate service delivery, rather than rely solely on the infrastructure of the health system (Aylward and Linkins 2005).

Looking Forward: How Best to Exploit the Lessons Learned?

The GPEI's late stage challenges have shattered any illusions that the implementation and success of future eradication efforts will be straightforward and largely predictable once the classical "feasibility" criteria have been met. However, just as with the lessons from smallpox eradication (Fenner et al. 1988), the lessons from the GPEI will have variable utility for most future eradication initiatives, depending on the nature of those efforts and the periods in which they are pursued (Cochi et al. 1998). Furthermore, much of the wealth of the GPEI's lessons will never be captured in textbooks or academic articles because many of the details, especially with regard to what didn't work, will survive only in the knowledge and experience of the thousands of individuals who worked at the various levels of this global initiative, often for more than a decade. Such "soft" or "tacit" knowledge will eventually dissipate as quickly as the GPEI's hard, physical resources will deteriorate in the tropical climates where they are concentrated. Consequently, the opportunity to exploit these lessons fully may be both time-limited and initiative-specific.

For these reasons, as well as the potential for cost-sharing, cost reductions, and efficiencies, it has been argued that the final phase of the GPEI should be merged or overlapped with a measles eradication initiative. This, it is argued, could exploit the GPEI's extensive human and physical infrastructure and ensure the hard lessons recently learned through the GPEI, especially in operations management, are optimally and effectively utilized. At the end of 2010, however, other commentators were arguing equally vociferously that the GPEI must be completed (successfully) before deciding on, let alone launching, a new eradication effort. While this perspective also has real merit, if there is to be a measles eradication initiative at some point in the future, it could be appropriate to consider merging or overlapping it with the final phase of the GPEI so as to avoid inadvertently increasing the costs and reducing the program's efficiency.

Whether a case can be made for concurrent eradication initiatives in the future will depend a great deal on the nature of each effort. In the case of measles and polio, however, the real choice may be whether to merge a measles eradication effort with the final phase of the GPEI or to risk foregoing measles eradication altogether, at least in the foreseeable future. The "win-win" rationale for combining these particular initiatives is rather straightforward:

First, once the GPEI interrupts wild poliovirus transmission globally, it will still need to sustain much of its core human and physical infrastructure for at least 6–8 years to facilitate certification of eradication, coordinate the eventual cessation of OPV use globally, and then verify the elimination of any residual vaccine-derived polioviruses (Aylward et al. 2006) (Figure 2.5).

Second, due to the reduced frequency of OPV campaigns during this period, there will be substantial excess capacity in this infrastructure which has most of the skills, knowledge, and geographic coverage needed for a measles eradication effort.

Third, once wild poliovirus transmission is interrupted, it may be easier to sustain GPEI financing and support, especially for resource-poor areas, if integrated with another initiative to address an important cause of childhood morbidity and, in the case of measles, mortality.

Finally, even if a measles eradication initiative were to ultimately prove unsuccessful, an intensified immunization and surveillance effort against the disease, integrated with the final phase of the GPEI, should be highly cost-effective in itself, especially as the use of the GPEI's infrastructure might reduce costs by as much as 30%.

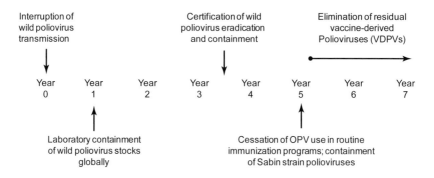

Figure 2.5   Timeline for the management of residual poliovirus risks following the eradication of wild type viruses globally.

impact in reducing measles incidence in the region (Figure 3.1). Following the catch-up campaign in the English-speaking Caribbean in 1991, it has been more than 14 years since the last indigenous laboratory-confirmed case was reported from those countries. Similarly, it has been more than 17 years since the last laboratory-confirmed measles case was detected in Cuba (Andrus et al. 2011a). As a direct result of these successes, as well as the eradication of poliomyelitis from the Americas, in September 1994 the Ministers of Health of the Region of the Americas unanimously established the goal of measles eradication from the Western Hemisphere by 2000.

Nearly all countries had eliminated endemic measles disease by the target date of 2000. However, in 2001–2002 a huge measles outbreak occurred in Colombia and Venezuela, resulting from a measles virus importation from Europe. Transmission of the imported virus D9 genotype was stopped with supplemental immunization campaigns in November 2002. This outbreak most likely represents the last endemic transmission in the region. The damage caused by the outbreak was substantial. During this outbreak, Colombia and Venezuela reported 139 and 2501 measles cases, respectively (Andrus et al. 2010).

Beginning in 2003, Mexico experienced an outbreak that resulted from an importation of measles virus H1 genotype. This particular genotype had never been previously isolated in the Americas, but is quite common in the Far East. Because population immunity was high, the outbreak remained relatively small and contained. From April 2003 to July 2004, a total of 108 measles cases were reported with all but two cases occurring in the contiguous two states and Federal District of Mexico City (Andrus et al. 2011a).

From February 2006 to February 2007, Venezuela reported 122 cases following an importation, which quickly became the largest of all measles

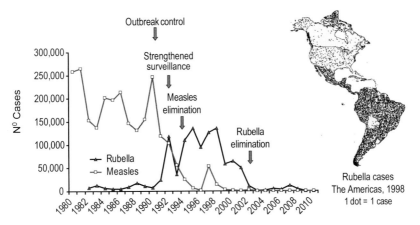

Figure 3.1   Reported measles and rubella cases in the Americas from 1980–2010. Source: EPI tables (1999–2003) and country reports to PAHO/WHO (since 2004).

outbreaks in the post-elimination era. Three distinct foci occurred in the outbreak. Active case searches conducted during a previously silent period of zero reporting of cases (between epidemiological weeks 27 and 43, 2006) identified 14 cases that had not been previously reported. The viruses identified for all three foci were all genotype B3 (de Quadros et al. 2008).

Importations are to be expected to be the norm if endemic transmission is still occurring in other parts of the world. The PAHO strategy has clearly demonstrated that regional measles eradication is indeed possible, particularly when the strategies are implemented well. But can it be sustained?

Fortunately, PAHO advised countries early on to incorporate rubella vaccine into their routine immunization programs. This action provided a foundation of population immunity through the use of measles–rubella (MR) or measles–mumps–rubella (MMR) vaccines, upon which additional tactics could be constructed to achieve the eradication of rubella and congenital rubella syndrome (Andrus et al. 2006).

Rubella and Congenital Rubella Syndrome Eradication Sustains Measles Eradication

Active measles surveillance unveiled the hidden disease burden of rubella and congenital rubella syndrome in the Americas (Figure 3.1). In September 2003, PAHO adopted a target for rubella elimination by 2010 (PAHO 2003). Prior to 2003, PAHO recommended that vaccines used in all measles vaccination strategies contain rubella as a component either as MR or MMR. The aim was to avoid missing an opportunity to control another serious public health threat and to provide support for other essential health services (Andrus and Roses Periago 2004; Castillo-Solórzano and Andrus 2004). As a result of accelerated integrated measles and rubella surveillance, experts estimated that approximately 20,000 congenital rubella syndrome cases (CRS) were occurring annually in the countries of Latin America and the Caribbean (Andrus et al. 2006) prior to the large-scale introduction of rubella-containing vaccine. The magnitude of the CRS problem prior to measles eradication had been largely unknown.

The eradication of rubella and CRS requires the thorough and rapid vaccination of adults to reduce the numbers of susceptibles in older populations and thereby, the continuing circulation of the virus (Andrus et al. 2006). Therefore, large, one-time "speed-up" mass rubella vaccination campaigns were implemented in all countries, targeting both women and men age <40 years using MR vaccine. In most countries the target group represented approximately 45% of the nation's population. These efforts were a huge undertaking, but experience demonstrated that if done well, only one campaign was required to interrupt endemic rubella transmission (Castillo-Solórzano and de Quadros 2002). The added benefit of using MR vaccine is that it boosted measles

population immunity and so protected the country from both measles and rubella importations and their spread. Rigorous analysis of the surveillance and
vaccination coverage data determined within each country the effectiveness of
the campaign.

The molecular epidemiology data indicate that the last endemic case of
measles in the region was in November 2002 (Figure 3.2). All other virus isolates in subsequent years are a result of importations from the rest of the world.
To support country commitment to maintain their measles and rubella eradication status, PAHO has mandated that transmission occurring in a LAC country
as a result of virus importation that lasts more than a year should be considered
endemic transmission, and that such a country would no longer be considered
as having eradicated these diseases (PAHO 2004).

Critical to maintaining the achievement of measles and rubella elimination
has been sustaining high-quality surveillance, and maintaining high levels of
population immunity with high routine measles coverage and the continued
implementation of "follow-up" campaigns with MR vaccine every four years.
In so doing, importations, once they occur, are contained much more effectively with rapid interruption of transmission (Castillo-Solórzano et al. 2008).
Cumulative global knowledge regarding the molecular epidemiology of rubella virus transmission is increasing rapidly, enabling the region of the Americas
to more readily determine which virus isolates are endemic and which are imported. In particular, a substantial number of rubella virus genotypes have been
detected throughout the Americas, with the most common ones including 1 B,
1C, 1E, and 2B genotypes. These virologic data are critical evidence to document that measles and rubella eradication are being sustained.

Lessons Learned and Implications for the Future

The routine national immunization programs in the Americas spearheaded the
eradication of polio, measles, rubella, and congenital rubella syndrome. The
strengthened routine immunization program served all in the public sector and
permitted the initiation and expansion of other programs to control vaccine-
preventable diseases. The prime objective has always been to target the most
vulnerable populations using the data from coverage performance and surveillance. One important by-product of this approach has been the strengthened
capacity for countries to introduce new life-saving vaccines, as well as respond
to emergencies (Andrus et al. 2010). In 2004, only 13 countries had introduced
seasonal influenza vaccination. Today, more than 35 countries have introduced
seasonal influenza vaccination (Ropero-Alvarez et al. 2009). In addition, the
number of LAC countries that have introduced pneumococcal conjugate, rotavirus, and HPV vaccines are 16, 16, and 6, respectively. Countries have been
able to reduce the time lag between the development of new vaccines and their
introduction into use in the developing countries.

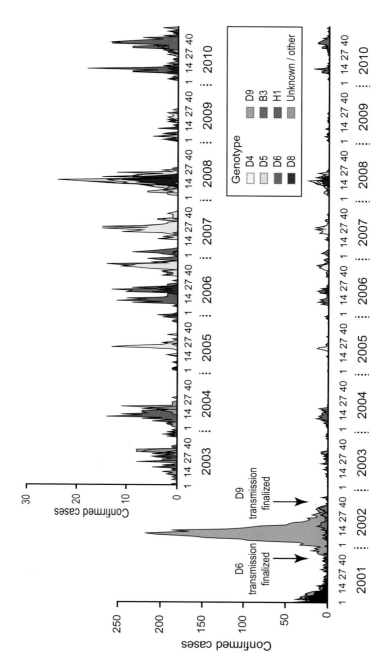

Figure 3.2 Reported measles cases in the Americas from 2001–2010 (bottom), with magnification of confirmed cases from 2003–2010 shown in the top panel. Source: Country reports to FCH/IM Global Measles Laboratory. Note: Canadian cases from 2008 (D8 genotype) were linked to a case or transmission chain where the source of index case is unknown.

Evidence from Uruguay and Chile suggests that these countries may have eliminated invasive *Haemophilus influenzae* type b (Hib) disease (Danovaro-Holiday et al. 2008). Coverage for this vaccine is generally >90% in all countries throughout the region. Experience in the United States and Canada suggests that when such coverage is achieved, the disease disappears. To that end, PAHO is mobilizing resources to better document this achievement. One important by-product will be strengthened surveillance. This experience and the data should help countries in other regions with their policy decisions on the potential introduction of Hib vaccine.

The accelerated introduction and deployment of new vaccines, and the potential elimination of invasive Hib disease, would not have been possible if routine immunization had not been prioritized as a critical public health function in the developing countries of the Americas, taking precedence over the short-term disease eradication initiatives. However, the short-term eradication initiatives served to provide a special influx of enthusiasm, commitment, and solidarity for national immunization programs.

Conclusions

The challenge for regions embarking on strategies similar to PAHO's strategy will be to maintain high population immunity with excellent immunization coverage and high-quality surveillance, especially to deal with importations. In addition, implementation of measles eradication strategies uncovered the "hidden" disease burden of rubella and CRS.

The last endemic case of measles in the Americas was reported in 2002, and the last endemic case of rubella in 2009. Meanwhile, substantial progress has been achieved in accelerating introduction and deployment of new vaccines in populations who need them most (Andrus et al. 2009). Integrating the eradication of measles with the eradication of rubella has greatly enhanced the capacity of countries to sustain progress. Such efforts have fostered a culture of prevention among adult men and women and have served as a springboard for the transition from child to family immunization programs (Tambini et al. 2006). In addition, countries are encountering new opportunities to expand the benefits of disease control and elimination activities to other aspects of public health, most importantly in improving health care for women and reducing inequities in health care in the poorest countries (Andrus and Roses Periago 2004; Castillo-Solórzano and Andrus 2004; Andrus et al. 2009). It is expected that the adoption of similar strategies in countries worldwide would achieve global eradication of measles in the next decade of the twenty-first century (Andrus et al. 2011b).

4

Onchocerciasis: From Control to Possible Eradication

Adrian Hopkins

Abstract

Our understanding of onchocerciasis has evolved over the last one and a half centuries from a description of an annoying skin disease, called aptly enough "craw craw," to an understanding of its transmission cycle and important role in blindness. Various control measures have been instituted as new tools have become available, and these have moved the field toward elimination and possible eradication. A review of the evolution of the program and the lessons learned along the way may be beneficial to other disease programs as they begin the "long march to elimination"—a journey that seems to speed up as the end draws near, but which is made difficult by last remaining cases and the enormous efforts these require to address.

Introduction

The first lesson to learn in any war is to know the enemy. Onchocerciasis was first described in Ghana, where the intense itching and associated skin changes were given a local name of "craw craw" (Figure 4.1). O'Neil (1875) first described the presence of filaria in the skin of those infected. Robels (1917) described a similar disease in the Americas. The relationship with the black fly vector was demonstrated by Blacklock (1926), but the relationship to blindness was a bit more controversial. Hissette (1932) first described the effects of the microfilaria on the eye in the Belgian Congo, with Ridley (1945) fully describing the eye signs in what is now Ghana. As the basic disease pattern and method of transmission became better understood, it was clear that there were many variations. In Africa, there is a difference between the more blinding form of savannah onchocerciasis and its vectors and the forest form and its vectors (Duke and Anderson 1972; Duke and Garner 1976). In the Americas, the parasite is similar to the West African species and was probably brought over during slave trade (Zimmerman et al. 1994). However, the simulium vector is different, and it also differs between the various foci. In Africa the vectors

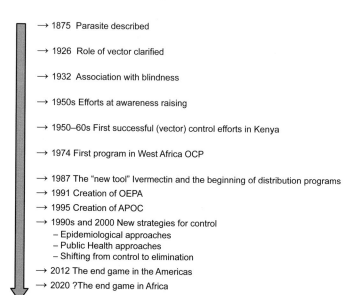

→ 1875 Parasite described

→ 1926 Role of vector clarified

→ 1932 Association with blindness

→ 1950s Efforts at awareness raising

→ 1950–60s First successful (vector) control efforts in Kenya

→ 1974 First program in West Africa OCP

→ 1987 The "new tool" Ivermectin and the beginning of distribution programs
→ 1991 Creation of OEPA
→ 1995 Creation of APOC
→ 1990s and 2000 New strategies for control
  – Epidemiological approaches
  – Public Health approaches
  – Shifting from control to elimination
→ 2012 The end game in the Americas
→ 2020 ?The end game in Africa

Figure 4.1   Time line of efforts to eliminate onchocerciasis.

are again very different: some have potential long flight ranges while others are very short. Understanding vector movements as well as the disease foci is essential for the programs to succeed. However, understanding the disease (and its vectors) is not enough to begin a control/elimination program. This chapter reviews the evolution of the onchocerciasis program and the lessons learned along the way, which could be useful as other disease programs begin the long march to elimination or eradication where the last cases will take enormous efforts.

Advocacy

Creating awareness of a disease among medical and public health authorities and the general public is an essential step toward control. When Sir John Wilson (founder of the British Empire Society for the Blind, now known as Sightsavers) visited Ghana with his wife, Jean, in 1946, they realized firsthand the impact of the disease, both as a public health and a personal problem. Stuck in their vehicle in a riverbed with all the windows closed to avoid simulium bites, Jean remarked to Sir John (Coles 2006:50):

> You know, it's no good calling this thing onchocerciasis. No one can pronounce it or spell it. You certainly can't raise funds for it. Let's call it "river blindness."

Since its establishment in 1950, Sightsavers has conducted research into onchocerciasis to back up their advocacy and to advance control (Crisp 1956).

Advocacy is not a singular event to get a program going. As new tools become available, as new strategies develop, and as control changes to an elimination or eradication initiative, continuous feedback must be supplied to the political, funding, and scientific communities. The two major onchocerciasis programs—the Onchocerciasis Elimination Program for the Americas (OEPA) and the African Program for Onchocerciasis Control (APOC)—have been very effective in advocacy, publishing results and keeping in regular contact with their donors to inform them of progress. The former Onchocerciasis Control Program (OCP), which covered a large area of West Africa, was also very effective in generating support. In fact, some of the original funding partners of OCP, when it was launched in 1974, are still active.

Program Issues

Develop Strategies Based on Wide-Ranging Scientific Disciplines

Successful elimination/eradication programs require a full understanding of the basic science around the disease agent and its vector, as well as the strategies to be applied. The OCP strategy involved vector control: insecticides were deposited in rivers to target breeding sites. This strategy was first established in Kenya (Roberts et al. 1986), where the vector was relatively easy to control, before the danger of dumping harmful insecticides in the environment was fully understood. OCP control policy required regular deposition of an approved insecticide on breeding sites with close monitoring of insecticide resistance and possible adverse effects on the flora and fauna (Samba 1994; Boatin 2008). One interesting aspect of the program involves the public's perception of noninfected flies, which returned following the cessation of vector control; in some areas, the local population believed that the program failed because the flies returned. This highlights the importance of informing the population fully to ensure that they understand the process. Detailed social and anthropological surveys may be required to construct appropriate messages throughout the program.

The major change in onchocerciasis control occurred in 1987, when Merck and Co., Inc. announced the donation of Mectizan® (ivermectin) to as many people as needed it for as long as it was required. This was the first effort to attack the parasite itself. However, while fully effective against the larva (microfilaria), Mectizan® is only partially effective against the adult worm. Initially, it was given to communities in a very controlled manner and to individuals under treatment by physicians. Strategies changed as knowledge grew about the safety and efficacy of Mectizan®. By the early 1990s, many of the worst affected communities were already receiving mass treatment, and it was understood that treatment would be required for some years. Initially, ten years was the timeframe thought to be sufficient; however, as experience increased, computer modeling indicated that twenty years would be more realistic, depending on initial prevalence and drug coverage. At the initial stages of the control program, it was noted that hypoendemic communities did not suffer much from either blindness or skin problems and were thus excluded; only more severely affected communities received treatment. Mobilizing communities for a 20-year control program required not only a good mechanism to determine which communities should be treated, but also methods to work with these communities to maintain momentum. The social sciences proved to be an essential part of ongoing program development. Now as strategies are turning toward elimination, some of those early decisions may need to be reconsidered. Because transmission is ongoing in some hypoendemic areas, treatment areas are being redefined as "transmission zones." Some areas which have achieved good coverage seem now to be clear of the disease with current treatment. In-country human capacity must be developed to clarify the epidemiological status and to maintain surveillance. Problem areas (e.g., co-endemic areas with loiasis and onchocerciasis) become increasingly important when the goal is elimination/eradication. Different or modified strategies may be required (i.e., twice yearly rather than annual treatment with Mectizan®). As control shifts to elimination, ongoing research in a variety of disciplines is imperative so that the best strategies can be developed.

Develop Broad-Based Partnerships

The impetus for an eradication program may initially come from a few committed scientists, but moving to the implementation phase requires a broad-based partnership, including representatives of the various scientific disciplines involved, public health experts, social scientists, and funding organizations. Nongovernmental organizations also play a crucial role by partnering with Ministries of Health to implement different control or eradication strategies. Partnerships require nurturing. When different partners are committed to the same overall objective, distinct priorities can be harmonized and everyone will benefit from the various insights each partner brings to the table. The success of the APOC program was highlighted during the annual Joint Action Forum in December 2010 (World Bank/APOC 2010):

> APOC, established in 1995, brings together 19 African countries affected by river blindness in an effort to control and where possible, eliminate, this neglected tropical disease (NTD). APOC is led by the World Health Organization through technical and managerial support from program headquarters in Burkina Faso. As the longest running public-private partnership for health in Africa, APOC is unique in the involvement of a broad range of financial, scientific and operational partners. With strong leadership from African ministries of health and support from 146,000 local communities and some 15 international non-governmental organizations, APOC provided nearly 70 million people with treatment for river blindness in 2009.

Involve the Communities in the Process

All elimination programs target communities, yet the level of community involvement has been highly variable. Some programs regard the public as passive recipients of what is deemed to be "good for them" by those who know. When the community does not want to be treated in such a way, this has sometimes been met with surprise.

To inform the community and mobilize the population for implementation, many programs use volunteers from the community. In some programs, volunteers are well paid for the few days' work that must be completed for each treatment cycle. Although paying volunteers may be useful for quick interventions, it is clearly not a viable option for onchocerciasis control because Mectizan® must be distributed over a period of many years.

Various community approaches have been attempted with increasing responsibility given to the community. Research by APOC with the Special Programme for Research & Training in Tropical Diseases (TDR) shows that communities fully empowered to take their own initiatives are completely able to carry out Mectizan® distribution at the community level. This has led to the development of community-directed treatment with ivermectin or CDTI (Homeida et al. 2002; APOC 2009). The CDTI approach has been extended to other health interventions and, for some mass interventions, community-directed interventions (CDIs) have proved to be highly effective in terms of coverage as well as sustainability (WHO/TDR 2008).

Integrate with the Health System

Some purely vertical targeted, short-term programs may be effective, but most eradication programs move from a control phase to an eradication initiative over a period of time, as have the onchocerciasis control programs. As initiatives progress over a longer timeframe, the specific strategies of an eradication program need to be integrated into the primary health care system at all levels, most importantly at the peripheral level.

The health care workers in charge of health centers are the key coordinators and the interface between the health system and the community. Some onchocerciasis control programs have run almost parallel programs, which becomes a problem when complications arise or where programs are not getting optimal results. Peripheral health workers are also responsible for the early reporting of cases.

The connection between the specifics of a vertical approach and the need for a horizontal implementation approach has led to what is sometimes described as a diagonal approach (A. D. Hopkins 2009). When programs are not fully integrated into the health system, financial sustainability and technical and logistical support become difficult to maintain (Gyapong et al. 2010). Where programs are well integrated into primary health care, there is good evidence to support the idea that health systems are strengthened from the "bottom up" (WHO/APOC 2007a). One way to help the process is to get the national health information systems to collect the data for whatever indicators are used. Peripheral health staff, who have to fill in a slot in their statistics sheets, are more likely to understand the importance of the activity.

Continue with Operational Research as Issues Arise

As programs transform from control to eventual elimination or eradication, new issues require study to increase the effectiveness of the various activities. One aspect in all three major onchocerciasis control/elimination programs has been the operational research undertaken to resolve issues as they arise. With OCP, this was particularly related to the best use of insecticides for vector control, especially when resistance began to be an issue. It was operational research that developed the rapid mapping of the disease (Ngoumou and Wash 1993) and the CDTI approach for the APOC program, but it has also addressed other issues (e.g., various possibilities for co-implementation, new issues around transmission zones, and modalities of treatment in the pipeline).

Modeling the disease is an ongoing process that requires continual updating as more information becomes available. In the OEPA countries, smaller foci have enabled very detailed ophthalmological, parasitological, and entomological data to be collected regularly, and this has been the basis of all program decision making (Sauerbrey 2008).

As the program moves forward, some of the research topics that will need attention include changes in the criteria for treatment and improved diagnostics, particularly for knowing when to stop (WHO/APOC 2009).

Fix Targets but Be Flexible

A 2003 conference concluded that onchocerciasis could be eliminated in the Americas but that elimination was unlikely to be achieved in Africa, apart from certain foci (Dadzie et al. 2003). A target was set to eliminate onchocerciasis by 2012 in the Americas. In Africa, the focus was put on building up to high, widespread coverage in meso- and hyperendemic areas to eliminate the disease "as a public health problem" (i.e., to control the worst effects of the disease in the most affected communities). From programs that had conducted longstanding ivermectin distribution in Africa, and as a result of studies which showed that transmission of the disease had been eliminated in some areas of West Africa (Diawara et al. 2009), questions surfaced as to "when treatment could be stopped."

The APOC mandate is evolving from establishing sustainable ivermectin distribution systems in all meso- and hyperendemic areas by 2015 to eliminating onchocerciasis, where possible, within the same time period. At the APOC Joint Action Forum in December 2010, it was proposed that an extension of

APOC could result in the elimination of transmission in most African countries by 2020.

Final Stages Will Be More Difficult and Costly

Control programs tend to begin in the easiest places to ensure that good results are accomplished. The APOC program began in areas where nongovernmental development organizations (NGDOs) had already been working and was thus able to be established on top of existing projects. This, together with the CDTI strategy, permitted a massive and effective scale-up in numbers of people under effective control.

However, repeated conflict in the D. R. Congo, southern Sudan, the Central African Republic, and Angola has hindered the scale-up of the APOC program in these conflict and post-conflict countries (WHO/APOC 2007a). The last places to be cleared of onchocerciasis will be those areas where work is most difficult, where the infrastructure has been destroyed, where qualified human resources are in scarce supply, and only limited national funding resources are available for the health system. These places will most likely pose some of the biggest difficulties to achieving the high coverage needed with ivermectin. As control moves to elimination, new strategies may be needed for these problem areas. As programs focus on the final remaining communities, which are usually in remote areas, follow-up will, once again, pose logistical difficulties and be comparatively very expensive to complete.

Keep Stakeholders Engaged

The partners involved in APOC are often referred to as the "APOC family." The World Bank, which is the fiscal agent for the trust fund, makes certain that all partners are kept informed, not just at the Joint Action Forum—when the whole "family" is convened—but also during the rest of the year (World Bank 2011a). The success of this engagement of partners contributing to the trust fund can be traced back to the OCP program in the 1970s; since then, many partners have contributed on a regular basis.

The APOC family depends on the major contribution of donated Mectizan®, without which there would be no APOC, government support and the involvement of NGDOs, which contribute up to 25%, and technical assistance where required (Haddad et al. 2008). This partnership requires transparency, openness, and a share in the successes. Like all families, disagreements arise from time to time over which strategies are best, but frank discussion and a steadfast commitment to the common final goal keeps the coalition strong and helps maintain progress.

Monitoring, Evaluation, and Surveillance

The advantage of the onchocerciasis program can be found in the method of control: following a simple dosing regimen, mass drug administration (MDA) of a safe drug is used and there are few side effects. Because the drug is so safe, the trigger point for beginning a control treatment has been considerably simplified. As MDA for onchocerciasis is integrated into the preventive chemotherapy (PCT) program of WHO (2006c), as well as the integrated monitoring of PCT programs, care must be taken to ensure that the specifics of onchocerciasis eradication are not lost in a mass of tablet distribution.

Baseline

REMO mapping (or rapid epidemiological mapping of onchocerciasis) is a tool used to determine where to treat. It is not, however, a full pretreatment epidemiological evaluation. As programs move toward the goal of eradication, it will be necessary to redefine these areas and collect solid epidemiological information on which to base decisions about stopping treatment. APOC countries will also need to train local national staff to carry out these parasitological and entomological surveys. In the lymphatic filariasis program, mapping using immunochromatography (ICT) cards has always been backed up by epidemiological surveys, which must be conducted before treatment can begin.

Coverage Figures

To move from control to elimination requires a high level of MDA coverage. APOC's target is 80% of the total population, which equates to over 90% of the eligible population, because children under 5 years of age, women who are pregnant or lactating during the first post-delivery week, and those who are chronically ill are not eligible for treatment. MDA is done by community distributors who establish their own registers of the population. Independent monitoring does happen in projects from time to time, but there are no regular post-treatment coverage surveys to monitor the work of the distributors, although techniques are available (Schwarz et al. 1999). In Ghana, significant population growth in some areas has led to the formation of new communities or "sub-villages." Community distributors have only counted and treated the initial villages in their program, leaving these new communities without MDA, and not included in the coverage calculation leading to an artificially high coverage figure. The lymphatic filariasis program, in contrast, has a formalized annual reporting system. For NTDs, WHO has developed guidelines to help monitor treatment coverage (WHO 2010d).

Diagnostic Tools

When the program goal was control, impact was measured in terms of morbidity, prevalence of visual impairment and blindness, and prevalence of debilitating skin disease. As the program evolves from control to elimination/eradication, more specific and sensitive diagnostic tools are required. One possibility with onchocerciasis is to test the flies, if these can be caught and analyzed easily. Using human flycatchers, however, is getting more difficult, both from a practical and ethical standpoint.

Populations are becoming more resistant to skin snips, which, although considered in some ways the "gold standard," are actually not very sensitive when there is a low prevalence of the disease. APOC is using the DEC (diethylcarbamazine) patch test, which since the early trials has developed into a more practical tool, but still has problems of reliability. The OEPA uses the OV16 antibody test, which is only useful for patients who have never been infected and thus must be targeted toward children. At present, there is no ideal test, and it remains to be determined how much research should be done to ensure that there are no new infections.

What Constitutes Eradication? What Number Is Zero?

The emphasis for onchocerciasis eradication has been the "elimination of transmission." There is a point at which the disease is no longer able to reproduce itself. In onchocerciasis eradication models, this is termed the breakpoint and has led APOC to define "elimination" as follows:

Elimination occurs when:

- Interventions in a defined geographical area have reduced *Onchocerca volvulus* infection and transmission to a point where the parasite population is believed to be irreversibly moving to its demise or extinction (i.e., below the breakpoint).
- Interventions at that point have been stopped.
- Post-intervention surveillance for an appropriate period has demonstrated no recrudescence of transmission to a level suggesting recovery of the *O. volvulus* population.
- Additional surveillance is necessary for timely detection of reintroduced infection from other areas.

Eradication of onchocerciasis will only occur when all old cases are no longer infected. This will happen when transmission is interrupted for a long enough time, but will not fit into this definition initially.

In 2000, the WHO defined elimination of onchocerciasis using criteria of morbidity (defined as the absence of microfilariae in the anterior segment of the eye) and transmission criteria defined as:

- OCP standard of infective larvae (L3) in flies <0.05% (0.1% in parous flies),
- annual transmission potential lower than 5–20 L3 per season,
- absence of detectable infection in school children and an antibody prevalence of <0.1%, and finally
- no new infections in recent migrants.

These criteria, however, do not fit all circumstances due to differences in the vector and the epidemiology.

Conclusion

Over the past half century, onchocerciasis control has progressed from the strategy of vector control to strategies based on mass drug administration. Success of the current strategies and the strong cooperation of affected communities have altered the vision from one of disease control to interruption of transmission within the next ten years and eventual eradication. The tasks ahead are to meet the current elimination goals and develop the surveillance, monitoring, and diagnostic tools that make it possible to certify that the disease has been eradicated.

Critical Issues in Determining Feasibility of Eradication

5

Political and Social Determinants of Disease Eradication

Robert G. Hall

Abstract

Eradication of disease is a major social achievement. To date, six attempts have been made to eradicate diseases in which humans are the primary or sole host, but only one has been successful. Success depends on very high levels of participation, beyond the levels predicted if individual community members act rationally in a self-interested way. Because near-universal participation is a condition of the achievement of eradication, a global eradication initiative can be held to ransom by a single country or small political groups. It is not always in the interests of a country to participate in an eradication initiative, particularly if there are pressing health needs in other areas. Game theory provides a useful way of understanding these processes. To achieve disease eradication, an international system of diplomatic and financial incentives and enforcements will need to be developed.

Introduction

The eradication of an important disease is a pinnacle of collective human achievement, let alone of public health. The ability to free all future generations across the globe from the threat of death and disability from a disease ranks as one of the greatest contributions that can be made by social effort. Disease eradication brings large, multiple, and long-lasting benefits, improving both quantity and quality of life, bringing economic benefit, and political credit to those who directed the effort. The eradication of smallpox, for instance, has been responsible for a major improvement in health in nearly every country, with economic gain due to a vastly reduced need for control measures and a complete end to the costs of treating and caring for people with smallpox. The eradication of smallpox conferred enormous political legitimacy on the

World Health Organization and other agencies which sponsored and directed the program. Indeed, the success of this effort has driven the search for other eradicable diseases and the development of proposals to initiate further disease eradication programs.

Eradication

As a concept, disease eradication appears to have first originated with Jenner, when he wrote in 1801 (Fenner et al. 1988:259):

> ...it now becomes too manifest to admit of controversy, that the annihilation of the Small Pox, the most dreadful scourge of the human species, must be the final result of this practice.

However, it was only in the 20th century that serious attempts were made to eradicate infectious diseases from humans (Aylward et al. 2000a; Taylor 2009). Six diseases have been targeted: yellow fever (1915–1977), yaws (1954–1967), malaria (1955–1969), smallpox (1955–1980), polio (1988–continuing), and dracunculiasis (1986–continuing). To date, only one of these six diseases, smallpox, has been eradicated.

Many attempts have been made to define disease eradication. A workshop on "Global Disease Elimination and Eradication as Public Health Strategies" in Atlanta in 1998 reviewed several definitions and concluded that eradication was the "[p]ermanent reduction to zero of the worldwide incidence of infection caused by a specific agent as the result of deliberate efforts; intervention measures are no longer needed" (Dowdle 1998). This definition echoes the conclusions reached in 1997 at another workshop on the "Eradication of Infectious Diseases" (Ottesen et al. 1998) and has broad currency in the field.

Thus defined, eradication essentially rests on the proposition that complete and permanent removal of the risk of acquiring disease is both necessary and sufficient. It implies global reach, or there would be some remaining risk arising from some geographical areas. However, without absolute and permanent extinction of the infectious agent, this condition does not hold, and neither does the corollary, that intervention measures are not required. If risk persists at any level, then control measures of some kind are still required, though they may be minor, especially in comparison with the Herculean effort needed to achieve eradication of a disease. The situation of smallpox illustrates this point: in 1978, after eradication, there was an outbreak of smallpox, including one death, sourced from a laboratory (Fenner et al. 1988) because this aspect of control was not adequate. Stocks of viable smallpox virus still exist, and stringent control must be, and is, maintained over them, while surveillance for smallpox continues. Once the eradication of wild poliovirus has been achieved, the need for continuing control measures will be a considerable and larger problem; there will be a need for a stringent laboratory containment regime, since it is possible to manufacture poliovirus in the laboratory from its constituent parts (Cello et al. 2002), and this ability is now irrevocably present.

For these reasons, it is unlikely that it will ever be possible to abandon all control measures for an "eradicated" disease. Since it is impossible to remove risk entirely, I shall define eradication as the reduction of incidence of a disease to zero cases per unit time through deliberate efforts, allowing the reduction of control measures to a level that is both low and the minimum possible.

There are two consequences of this argument: Control measures must be maintained in perpetuity, so costs must be viewed as infinite. Also, organizational and international arrangements under some kind of global public health agreement need to be established and maintained indefinitely.

The Feasibility of Eradication

Conventionally, the feasibility of eradication of a disease has been considered to be determined by biological and social and political criteria. For each candidate disease, criteria have been defined by the International Task Force on Disease Eradication (MMWR 1993; Hinman and Hopkins 1998) as:

1. Biological criteria
   a. Epidemiological vulnerability
   b. Effective practical interventions likely to achieve eradication
   c. Demonstrated feasibility
2. Social and political criteria
   d. A broad social perception of the importance of the disease
   e. A reasonable projected cost
   f. Synergy with other health system activities
   g. Necessity for eradication rather than control

These criteria are commonly accepted, but they underemphasize the importance of the social and political criteria (Aylward et al. 2000a; Shiffman 2006; Bhattacharya and Dasgupta 2009; Taylor 2009). Due to its absolute nature, eradication requires universal engagement of countries (Barrett 2004) and generally very high engagement of populations within countries.

The degree of social and national engagement required depends on the endemicity and infectivity of the disease. It is easier to eradicate a disease with very limited geographical or social spread and easier to eradicate a disease of low infectivity. Eradication of endemic disease is more difficult, because there are more infectives that are spread over a greater geographical area (Barrett 2004). For highly infectious diseases, the requirements for mobilization of countries and their populations are very high indeed, and there are major risks for failure if universal engagement is not achieved. Polio and smallpox have roughly the same degree of infectivity (Anderson and May 1991:70, 88); however, polio was endemic in 125 countries at the beginning of the Global Polio Eradication

Initiative in 1988, whereas smallpox was present in only 59 countries (Barrett and Hoel 2007) at the beginning of the smallpox eradication program in 1958. Smallpox was an ideal candidate for eradication, and its eradication has proved easier than that of polio.

For a vaccine-preventable disease, the degree of social engagement required to eradicate a disease can be modeled. To achieve eradication of a vaccine-preventable disease, the number of persons in the population susceptible to the disease must be below a threshold, which is determined by the infectivity of the disease in the community. For highly infectious diseases this threshold is itself rather low, and while not everyone needs to be immunized, a very high proportion of the population does need to participate in the immunization program. Individuals, communities, and nations assess their willingness to participate against a number of criteria, and eradication of disease may not be of value to them. Because near-universal participation is needed, there is great scope for gaming, and social groupings, and indeed nations, may use their power of veto to demand concessions before they will participate in the eradication initiative. This problem is magnified if the effectiveness of the vaccine is low, or if several doses are required, or the disease has several different immunotypes.

Eradication is an absolute concept and has been referred to as "extreme" public health (Barrett and Hoel 2003); it is a great gamble (Barrett 2009). As a public health strategy, attempts at eradication have a mixed history: three of the six attempts (yellow fever, yaws, malaria) failed, while two (polio and dracunculiasis) are still in progress and one (smallpox) has been successful (Taylor 2009). The polio eradication program was successful in 1999 in eradicating type 2 poliovirus, one of three serotypes of polio (Barrett 2004). Eradication as a strategy is vulnerable to failure at many points.

Rationale for Eradication

Humanitarian arguments feature very prominently in the reasons advanced in support of eradication iniatives. These arguments note the improvement in health that can be made by freeing the world from target diseases. The resolution of the World Health Assembly in 1988, which committed the World Health Organization to the eradication of polio, makes no mention of economics, either in terms of costs or benefits (World Health Assembly 1988). Its rationale appears to be purely humanitarian; however, it does recognize the importance of politics in reaching the goal. The resolution on the eradication of smallpox, adopted in 1958, argued the humanitarian case, but also stated the Assembly's view that the costs of eradication would be less than the costs of control, and that successful eradication would make expenditures on smallpox control and treatment redundant (Fenner et al. 1988:368).

Social and Political Determinants of Eradication

I shall describe the factors that affect the outcome of an eradication program as "determinants," in that these factors interact among themselves to influence the outcome, and no single determinant completely predicts the outcome. I shall categorize the social and political determinants of eradication as being broadly economic as well as social and political. I shall discuss the economic considerations only briefly, as part of the setting for the social determinants.

Economic Considerations

Eradication of a disease can be considered in economic terms as an investment, where an expenditure in the present reaps dividends into the future (Barrett and Hoel 2007). There are often diminishing returns on health expenditure, but for disease eradication this is not true. As control improves, there are diminishing returns, but when eradication is achieved there are very great returns indeed. For smallpox, the dividend was enormous. A one-time investment made for smallpox eradication in 1967 of USD 100 million saved about USD 1.35 billion per year, which, assuming a 3% discount rate, resulted in a benefit/cost ratio of ~150/1. The benefit/cost ratio for the incremental cost of eradicating polio in 1967 was even larger: ~450/1. The benefit to the United States alone was USD 5 billion (Barrett 2004; Barrett and Hoel 2007). Barrett and Hoel (2007) describe this as "an astonishingly good deal" for the world. Countries can be strongly motivated to participate in eradication by the promises of a great return on such investments and, more critically, de-motivated when the returns on investment are low or, in the case of failure, negative.

The Utility of Eradication

Economically, eradication is always better than continued efforts and expenditure on high-level control. If eradication is feasible then it is always to be preferred, and altering course to change the objective from eradication to control is not economically optimal (Thompson and Duintjer Tebbens 2007; Barrett and Hoel 2007). Eradication requires greater effort in the short run, but returns a bigger dividend over the long term; for control, this situation is reversed (Barrett 2004). For polio, this means that the world should be willing to pay yet more to achieve eradication. If we return to a situation of low control, the epidemiology will revert to the situation in the 1980s, but with a bigger world population. This constitutes a very strong economic and public health case for eradication now (Thompson and Duintjer Tebbens 2007).

The returns from investment in a disease eradication initiative over the long term are very large; however, they accrue into the future, and their valuation depends on countries' and people's time consistency of preferences. It is difficult for communities and countries to value the far distant future in the same

way as the present, and this becomes particularly important in political processes, which are generally characterized by short time horizons.

The economic benefits and costs of disease eradication are not uniformly
distributed over populations or countries. Countries with a high burden of disease may benefit more, but the cost structure of the health care system will also
influence policymakers' views. To take the example of polio, the return to the
world as a whole on investment in eradication has been found to be high (Khan
and Ehreth 2003; Duintjer Tebbens et al. 2011). However, there are differences
between high- and lower- and middle-income countries. If polio immunization
were discontinued, eradication would be a good investment for high-income
countries. Most of these countries, however, have made policy decisions to
continue polio vaccination after eradication for other reasons, and thus the return will not include savings due to cessation of immunization (Barrett and
Hoel 2007). For countries proposing to cease polio immunization after eradication, eradication becomes economically optimal if lifetime welfare costs of
paralytic polio exceed USD 60 to USD 250. Treatment costs in low-income
countries are about USD 420, and Barrett and Hoel (2007) conclude that eradication is the preferred strategy.

Competing Priorities

Eradication may be a worthwhile goal for any country, but the proposal cannot be considered in a vacuum since there are always competing proposals.
Eradication may be a good investment in the long run, but it may not be the
best alternative in the present. For many countries, eradication of a disease that
can be well controlled by immunization may be a low priority when placed
alongside the burden of other diseases. This is a current problem for polio
eradication. For many countries in Africa, for instance, polio is not a high priority in terms of reducing the burden of disease.

Social and Political Engagement

Public health is, by definition, a collective enterprise and is therefore, of necessity, political. Public health programs, and especially large, high-risk proposals
like eradication, attract attention from a range of political actors including international organizations (both diplomatic and nongovernment), nation-states,
and political groupings within nation-states (Taylor 2009). Disease eradication
programs, especially those that use immunization to achieve these ends, are
"deeply social and political phenomena" (Bhattacharya and Dasgupta 2009).
Because high coverage is needed, it is impossible to conduct an immunization
program without paying due consideration to the social and political context
within which it occurs. For disease eradication to happen, a threshold minimum of the population must be removed from risk, and for vaccine-preventable
diseases this means the population must be immune. Epidemiological theory

describes a minimum susceptible population size needed to sustain continued transmission, and this is always a very small proportion of the global population. For all practical purposes disease eradication "relies on absolute commitment among all engaged parties" (Taylor 2009); there must be very high social commitment to eradication within a country, and disease eradication cannot be achieved if even one small country does not participate in the program. This creates a major diplomatic challenge. It is difficult to organize consensus among nations, and difficult to organize consensus within nations, since, though the costs are very evident, no single group by itself benefits enough from eradication to campaign for it (Farchy 2005). This is a not uncommon problem in international relations, and there is a history of both successes and failures. Universal agreements on smallpox and containment of atmospheric ozone depletion have been achieved (Barrett 2006), but agreement has eluded international negotiators for other universal projects, such as nuclear disarmament and targets for reduction in emissions of carbon dioxide.

The Politics of Eradication

Lessons from smallpox eradication that can assist other eradication initiatives include the need for long-term, high-level political commitment (Fenner et al. 1988:1349) and the understanding that "societal and political considerations ultimately determine success" (Aylward et al. 2000a:1515). It is often said that if political commitment is obtained, disease control and eradication initiatives will be strengthened and immunization coverage will increase. However, it is difficult to describe exactly what "political will" entails in this context (Gauri and Khaleghian 2002), and this argument does not sufficiently recognize all the other factors that determine the performance of an eradication program.

Disease eradication is a very large strategic gamble (Barrett 2009), and risk of failure is a major political problem. Countries fear for sunk costs if the program is ultimately unsuccessful. These costs are incurred up to the point of acceptance of failure and are not recoverable; because disease control will have to be maintained, this leads to a loss of political legitimacy (Farchy 2005; Barrett 2006, 2009). Failure may have dire political consequences for governments and the international organizations that have sponsored the unsuccessful eradication attempt. Countries will not participate unless confident of success, and the benefit conferred by failure is small or zero.

Community Participation in Immunization Programs

Immunization programs that target the entire population depend on reliable demand for vaccination and effective supply. This is immediately a sociopolitical argument, as participation depends on the perceptions of disease and risk held by individuals in the community, and competing priorities (Taylor 2009). Eradication of vaccine-preventable diseases raises the stakes, requiring high, though not universal, immunization coverage. Directly transmitted communicable diseases can only be spread to persons who are susceptible to the disease. This is the rationale for immunization, since it reduces, often to very low levels, the probability of transmitting disease from an infective to a vaccinated individual. If the infective person makes contact with only susceptible persons, the degree of transmission of the disease will depend on the properties of the disease in that community. If the infective person makes contact with only vaccinated persons, who are therefore not susceptible, transmission does not occur. If there are both vaccinated and unvaccinated persons in the community, the sustainability of transmission depends on the properties of the disease in the community and on the average number of contacts made with unvaccinated persons. For a large population, a threshold proportion of effectively immunized persons can be derived. Mathematically this is given by:

$$v^* \geq 1 - \frac{1}{R_0}, \tag{5.1}$$

where v^* is the proportion effectively immunized and R_0 is the average number of secondary cases due to a single infective in a completely susceptible population (Smith 1964). Thus it is not, in principle, necessary to obtain universal immunity to eradicate a disease, and it is possible to accommodate a limited degree of nonparticipation.

Estimates of the threshold "herd" immunity required to eradicate various diseases have been made. The range for most of the potentially eradicable diseases is between 70% and 95% (Anderson and May 1991:88). However, a number of factors must modify this conclusion. Vaccines are not perfectly effective, many vaccines require multiple doses for efficacy, and several diseases have multiple immunotypes, each of which requires threshold coverage for eradication. For practical purposes it is necessary to engage nearly the entire population of a country in this effort.

Individuals in a completely "rational" community would participate in an immunization program up to the level where the perceived benefits for each individual outweigh the perceived risks. The principal benefits are protection from disease, whereas the risks are the adverse effects of the vaccine. A community behaving in this manner would participate to the point where the disutility of adverse effects is just balanced by the utility of protection (Fine and Clarkson 1986). However, protection (or risk of disease) is afforded not only by an individual's own acceptance of a vaccine, it is also determined by uptake of the vaccine throughout the rest of the community. The incidence of the disease is dependent on immunization coverage, which is in turn dependent on the sum of individuals' decisions to accept vaccination. Decisions of an individual would therefore depend in part on the decisions made by other community members (Bauch et al. 2003). Game theory was developed to investigate such eventualities and one can describe a "vaccination game." Under this theory, a game reaches a stable point at a Nash equilibrium, when all players have adopted the best strategy available, given the strategies adopted by other players. The behavior of real populations can be modeled, and in general observed behavior follows convergently stable Nash equilibria (Bauch and Earn 2004). In a convergently stable Nash equilibrium, the strategies players adopt converge to a single strategy, irrespective of strategies adopted by other players. For the vaccination game, the relative risk of adverse effects of vaccination is defined as $r \equiv \frac{r_v}{r_i}$, the risk due to the vaccine (r_v) divided by the risk due to infection (r_i). Persons who perceive that $r > 1$ (i.e., the vaccine is more risky than taking one's chances with the disease) would not participate in the vaccination program, whereas persons perceiving $0 < r < 1$ would see benefit in vaccination and would participate. On the assumption that the behavior is "rational," Bauch and Earn show that the proportion of the community taking up vaccination under a convergently stable Nash equilibrium is given by $P*$ where

$$P^* = 1 - \frac{1}{R_0(1-r)} < 1 - \frac{1}{R_0}. \qquad (5.2)$$

R_0 is again the average number of secondary cases attributable to a single infective in a completely susceptible population. Thus, under these assumptions, a "rational" community would never participate in an immunization program to the extent necessary to eradicate a disease (Bauch and Earn 2004; Farchy 2005).

Further insights may be gained from game theory into the effects of adverse publicity. It is not at all uncommon for the media to propagate scare stories about the alleged adverse effects of vaccines, with consequent, sometimes disastrous, loss of public confidence in the immunization program. On the basis of their analysis, Bauch and Earn expect that the community would be more likely to refuse immunization for highly infectious diseases, compared with diseases of lower transmissibility.

Furthermore, the impact of vaccine scares and education programs to counter them would be asymmetrical. Vaccine scares would lead to rapid reductions in vaccine uptake, but public education campaigns on the value of immunization designed to offset scare stories would produce slower increases in uptake, because increasing uptake by the community as a whole would reduce an individual's incentive to participate (Bauch and Earn 2004). Both of these effects seem to occur in practice.

The first consequence of this analysis is that to achieve sufficient immunization coverage for eradication to be successful, community members have to participate beyond the extent determined by "rational" self interest. The decision to participate may entail a positive valuation of the health of others in addition to one's own, and this may include other members of the present community, or for future members, particularly one's descendants. In addition, education and other campaigns designed to mitigate the effects of scare stories are critical, and can often take time. Thus consistency and persistence are required.

A possible strategy for overcoming community nonparticipation in a program is to make participation compulsory (Lahariya 2007). Immunization is quasi-compulsory in many countries, where school entry laws require a certificate of immunization (or in some countries a certificate of exemption). Compulsion, even forcible compulsion, has been described in some places during the smallpox eradication program (Greenough 1995; Bhattacharya and Dasgupta 2009).

In practice, eradication of a disease cannot be achieved without engagement and participation of the entire population; therefore, eradication programs require a greater focus than is usually given to marginalized groups (Taylor 2009). Participation of hard-to-reach subpopulations becomes a critical part of eradication initiatives and necessitates the development of novel ways to engage with these communities that differ from the approaches of more routine health services. For example, uptake of polio vaccine among the Moslem population in northern India has been low in the recent past compared with the Hindu population, and the eradication program has attempted to engage this community by relabeling it as "underserved," a language that avoids religion as a potential barrier to participation (Taylor 2009).

There is a conflict between the interests of the community as a whole and the individuals within it (Fine and Clarkson 1986; Taylor 2009). Generally, public health staff tend to adopt a technical-scientific paradigm, and consider the social and political requirements of program operation to be of secondary importance. This leads to an attitude that tolerates a subversion of rights for the "greater good" (Lahariya 2007; Taylor 2009). This is sometimes reinforced by the fact that many public health staff are government employees and operate in an environment that uses regulation extensively to achieve public health ends. Eradication of a disease relies on universal commitment, yet a community's perception of a focus on a single disease, with consequent scaling back of emphasis on other concerns, may result in disengagement. The community responds to different diseases in different ways, owing to their different natural histories and different means of treatment and control. The effort put into polio control, for example, is perceived by many in the community, and even by many in the public health community, as being disproportionate to the risk it poses (Gersovitz and Hammer 2003; Taylor 2009).

Scientifically trained public health staff (especially Westerners) often interpret nonparticipation in immunization programs as being religious in nature. Although religious belief may play a role, this interpretation is usually an oversimplification. Local political leaders often use immunization as a wedge, holding the program hostage to other concerns (Bhattacharya and Dasgupta 2009). Essentially, this strategy works because of the value differences between local people and program managers and advocates.

Participation of a population in an eradication initiative is determined by a complex mix of factors. Participation of "rationally" behaving individuals will never be sufficient to eradicate a disease; some other motivation must be brought to bear. This may be altruism, a sense of commitment to society or one's descendants, or compulsion. Different strategies will be more or less effective in different contexts. These considerations then raise major ethical issues that need to be addressed by the eradication program.

Program Management

Disease eradication requires an enormous, global effort. It is a high-risk proposition, as any one of very many factors could cause the entire enterprise to fail. Strong program management is therefore an essential condition for success. Surprisingly, however, there is a dearth of high-quality evidence on the impact of management on the effectiveness of immunization programs. A search of the literature by Ryman et al. (2008) revealed 11,500 papers published between 1975 and 2004. Of these, only 25 met quality criteria. Their results focused on strategies to bring immunization services closer to the community, communication to increase demand for immunization, changing practices at fixed sites, and using more innovative management practices, all of which resulted in increase in uptake and community engagement (Ryman et al. 2008).

A World Bank study examined predictors of immunization service performance at national level, reviewing published data to construct a model of predictors of national immunization performance (Gauri and Khaleghian 2002). The broad findings were that:

- Global policy significantly affected immunization coverage, with the Universal Childhood Immunization initiative, for example, being most likely responsible for a major increase in coverage in most countries.
- Involvement with international agencies, such as UNICEF or revolving funds, affected coverage positively but delayed uptake of new vaccines.
- Democratic governments were associated with lower immunization coverage, but not in low-income countries.
- Supply-side factors, such as quality of a country's institutions, affected coverage but several demand-side factors did not. Institutional quality was measured using an index available to the World Bank, and demand-side factors included national income, literacy, access to mass media, female participation in the labor force, and previous experience of disease outbreaks.

Gauri and Khaleghian (2002) emphasize that, in their opinion, this does not provide support for the establishment and support of autocratic regimes. However, the study does indicate that international support and broad indicators of management quality are associated with higher coverage, and these have been major foci of activity in the operation and management of eradication activities.

global and national nongovernment organizations and foundations and a wide variety of bilateral and multilateral international arrangements (Bhattacharya and Dasgupta 2009). The history of disease eradication to date has been sponsorship by an international organization and delivery by nation-states, with a consequent potential for conflict (Smith et al. 2004; Taylor 2009). As a diplomatic organization, the World Health Organization has to give primacy to nation-states, but where the authority of the state is weak, the capacity to deliver an eradication program may be problematic. Compared with the era of the smallpox eradication program, there are now many more international actors. There are more nation-states, often with an increasing number of powerful regional political entities as well as powerful nongovernment organizations. For example, in the past, global immunization policy was by and large determined by the WHO, but now the World Bank, the Bill & Melinda Gates Foundation, the Global Alliance for Vaccines and Immunization, and Rotary International all influence policy.

Availability of donor funding for communicable diseases control programs, including eradication initiatives, may be analyzed in terms of recipient need, provider interest, or global policy frameworks (Shiffman 2006). Donor funding is poorly related to burden of disease in recipient countries and often reflects perceptions of burden in donor countries (Shiffman 2006).

There are incentives for international cooperation (Thompson and Duintjer Tebbens 2008a), but experience and game theory demonstrate that some degree of enforcement may be required (Barrett 2004). International law has been important in communicable disease control, and the International Health Regulations were developed as one means of achieving cooperation (Lazcano-Ponce et al. 2005; Gainotti et al. 2008).

A partial solution to this may be diplomatic and financial. It is possible to exert diplomatic pressure for eradication initiatives, and the WHO itself has attempted this in Nigeria. Countries can be supported financially to eradicate disease, if the priority for the country is lower than the priority for aid donors.

Conclusions

Disease eradication presents unique benefits and novel challenges. It is a high-stakes game, demanding universal participation over a prolonged period, in an environment where the mechanisms to ensure participation are weak. Yet eradication has been achieved on one occasion, and smallpox has been removed as a global threat. In addition, large areas of the world have eliminated polio, measles, rabies, dracunculiasis, lymphatic filariasis, and even malaria.

Disease eradication cannot be achieved without a vision for the future. If a community takes only its present self-interest into account, participation in eradication initiatives will never be sufficient to reach this goal. The investment case for eradication is on behalf of future generations, and advocacy

Table 6.1 Unsuccessful disease eradication programs and the reasons for their failure (based on data from CDC 1993a; Henderson 1998).

Disease, date	Reasons for failure:	Research needed:
Hookworm, 1907	Mass treatment does not cure; it only decreases infection intensity so reinfection occurs	To understand transmission dynamics and drivers of infection
Yellow fever, 1915	Animal reservoir in nonhuman primates in forested areas	To understand transmission dynamics and drivers of infection
Yaws, 1955	No treatment was given to inapparent cases	To be able to diagnose all stages of disease important to ongoing transmission
	Some patients with overt disease were only partially treated, leading to relapse and ongoing transmission	To understand transmission dynamics and drivers of infection
	Premature withdrawal of disease-specific programs caused reemergence	
Malaria, 1955	Development of resistance in vectors and parasite	Monitoring of resistance in vectors and parasite for early detection
	Complicated and challenging vector ecology to control approaches	Into new chemotherapeutic options and insecticides
	Administrative shortcomings and increasing costs of program	To understand transmission dynamics and drivers of infection in different ecological settings to modify plan accordingly

When Theory Meets Data: Changing Targets and Program Goals

Ideally, initial program targets are based on the best data available at the time an elimination or eradication program is established. Through program monitoring, the data informing these decisions will increase over time. Multiple examples, from almost every program, demonstrate that the data set at the beginning does not resemble the data at the end.

In 2000, the target was set to eliminate lymphatic filariasis (LF) as a public health problem by 2020. Currently, large-scale, community-based drug distribution programs are underway in an expanding number of endemic countries. The community drug distribution program for LF reached 546 million people in 2009 and is arguably the largest public health program that has ever been conducted (Chu et al. 2010; Ottesen et al. 2008). The initial World Health Organization (WHO) strategy for the elimination of LF was based on the expectation that four to six rounds of mass drug administration at a community level could eliminate LF from that community. The original targets set in 2000 were based on modeling with available data (Gambhir et al. 2010). The program is now at its midpoint, with ten years remaining to complete the task. New modeling, based on data from sites in Asia and Africa that exhibit different vectors, vector densities, population density and other factors, has shown significant variation between sites, depending on the local transmission dynamics. One of the greatest challenges to a global program is to prepare for and react to this immense local diversity (Gambhir et al. 2010). The main interplay takes place between the vector and control of disease transmission; by addressing the vector directly (i.e., vector control) and/or reducing the parasite in the infected host, transmission can be interrupted by eliminating the pool of microfilaria for the vector to transmit. Operational research is currently underway to assess vectors, coverage, compliance, drug dosage and frequency, and end points to verify the success of elimination. All of this work needs to result in appropriate program changes for implementation, or the success of the program will be jeopardized.

One challenge to programs is that lessons from early successes can be misleading or not representative, as was observed in LF elimination initiatives in South Korea and Yemen. Although both countries provided early examples of successful elimination, and both countries had relatively limited disease in lower levels, only one used the WHO strategic approach in their programs. Due to the different epidemiology, South Korea relied on a screen-and-treat approach, which was feasible because of the localized disease distribution patterns in the country, instead of the WHO mass drug administration approach. Significant social and economic developments were also factors for success in South Korea, leading to improved housing and good vector control, which complemented the chemotherapeutic approach. From this example, two factors are significant. First, all models must be scrutinized in context of the local situation; disease transmission is always multifactorial, thus the approach will need to vary accordingly. Second, during a program, environmental and social changes can impact transmission; these changes should be sought and used to guide research questions during the lifetime of a program.

One Size Doesn't Fit All

A chief criticism of the early efforts in the 1950s in the malaria eradication initiative was the rigidity of the approach and the lack of accompanying research and learning. The malaria program had high levels of political commitment: the director of a national program reported directly to the head of the government in a fully vertical program that had its own staff and pay scales. This strength was offset, however, by a significant weakness: the programs did not generally involve any level of the community. Instead, they had detailed standardized operating procedures and worked under the assumption that all of the needed technology was available. Success relied solely on the strict application of the interventions according to plan, and research or learning was not incorporated into the plan. Ultimately, after significant investment of human and financial resources, this strategy failed.

The smallpox program learned from these mistakes and took a very different approach, working within the health system and engaging local communities as part of the program. Instead of having standard operating procedures, the smallpox project set broad goals and enabled flexibility and creativity in how these goals were achieved locally. Research was also included as part of the work, and during the program many new ideas were adopted: new tools were developed for vaccine delivery; field studies provided insight into epidemiology and transmission and were used to modify the approach; studies looked for animal reservoirs; and studies were conducted on the duration of vaccine efficacy (Henderson 1998). Ultimately, this flexible approach, which embraced research, led to the first successful eradication program.

Lack of a Baseline

One of the reasons cited for the failure of yaws elimination was the lack of pilot programs in critical geographic areas (Henderson 1998). This key feature is integral to the start and ongoing management of any elimination or eradication program. With yaws, excitement over a new tool prompted an effort to be initiated without a full plan or learning agenda in place. The new tool was injectable penicillin, which enabled yaws to be treated with a single injection (Henderson 1998; Narain et al. 2010). As encouraging as this was, there was no baseline data to form the basis of a plan for elimination. When a test was developed and serological surveys were conducted, a much larger number of subclinical infections were demonstrated; this led to the resurgence of disease in communities after the overt clinical cases were treated and reestablished transmission. Since there was no proof of cure diagnostic, some patients were insufficiently treated, which led to disease recurrence and reestablished transmission. This resurgence was exacerbated by the early withdrawal of disease-specific teams, which meant that early signs of reemerging infection went undetected. Henderson (1998) postulates that if this baseline work had been conducted, the elimination program might never have been attempted with the tools available at the time.

Monitoring and setting targets is difficult, if not impossible, without a solid or at least semisolid foundation. Prevalence of disease was used for the baseline to follow progress in leprosy and was defined as all people receiving treatment at a given moment over the total population. Leprosy is a disease that requires long-term treatment, and this means that as programs and treatment recommendations changed, the populations receiving treatment also changed. Consequently, prevalence was altered without actually providing a true indication of the program's success. Take, for example, the decrease in multibacillary multidrug therapy from 24 to 12 months. Although this effectively cut the number of patients by half and resulted in a significant decline in disease prevalence, it did not actually change the status of the disease. In addition, data on cases were collected and counted annually as of December 31. Thus data from patients on 6-month therapy with paucibacillary multidrug therapy or who received a single treatment for a single skin lesion were not included in the prevalence figures, resulting in data that did not truly reflect the progress or issues associated with the program. Incidence of new cases provides a better and more interesting measure. However, because of the long incubation period of leprosy, which ranges from 2–20 years, incidence is not an accurate measure of elimination; thus, some sort of screening is required. Interestingly, due to the definitions being used, many sites have eliminated leprosy even though new cases are still detected annually, as seen in South Africa (Lockwood and Suneetha 2005). A program needs to screen for relapse for up to five years after treatment, because of the slow-growing nature of the organism. This has not been fully addressed in global targets of the elimination program. Even today, debate continues and experts question whether leprosy should be targeted for elimination or more honestly tackled as an ongoing disease program (CDC 1993b; Lockwood and Suneetha 2005).

Lack of baseline data has also been cited in LF elimination and has limited the program's ability to learn. In an evaluation of the LF elimination programs from five country islands in the Pacific, only one country was able to provide useful data. All others used a convenience sample for their baseline data collection, which meant that this data could not be compared to the follow-up data after five rounds of mass drug administration. This information would have been very helpful in modeling and providing indicators for modifying programs that did not successfully meet the targets (Huppatz et al. 2009). Setting up sentinel sites for evaluation and research, particularly in early countries, could be very valuable, as early investment can prove extremely useful to later programming.

Elimination as a Public Health Problem

The phrase "elimination as a public health problem" is unclear in most, if not all, contexts. It has been a rallying tool to garner additional attention and resources to an area, but defining what a public health "problem" is and what indicators can be used to determine when something is no longer a "problem" is problematic. In addition, regardless of the programmatic target set, public health efforts must be maintained and sensitive surveillance and response must be continued if the target is anything less than complete elimination or eradication (Molyneux et al. 2004). In these cases, setting reasonable measurable targets that are subject to reevaluation and discussion through a carefully thought-out research agenda could help decrease the ambiguity and clarify reasonable end points.

There are many examples of where this has not been done and programs have suffered as a result. In leprosy, the target for elimination is 1 case in a population of 10,000. This is a figure that can be easily manipulated by choosing a different denominator. In 2001 the WHO, despite data to the contrary, declared that leprosy had been eliminated as a public health problem by including in the denominator the total population of all the countries who had reported at least one case. What does this target truly indicate? Leprosy transmission still occurs, and incidence of new cases has not decreased in many settings despite the progress in decreased prevalence (Lockwood and Suneetha 2005). The importance of 1 case per 10,000 population for disease transmission or program planning is not clear; thus the significance of reaching or not reaching this target seems to have little meaning programmatically, outside of declaring that it has been met.

Proving Zero to Define Success

Starting a program is frequently straightforward: to eliminate a disease, you detect cases and intervene to block transmission. Of course, this becomes much more complicated, as discussed above, when you need to ensure that you can detect all cases and all stages of infection, and either treat completely or prevent further transmission. The final challenge is to prove success: How do you prove a zero? How do you address confidence intervals? These questions quickly become important, and early sites where successful elimination has been achieved will likely differ (e.g., in terms of lower transmission, different socioeconomic or cultural considerations) from areas that enter later in a program. How do these factors affect indicators and measures of success?

All elimination or eradication programs struggle with these issues. The fact that we cannot prove a zero means that we need to find another way. This challenge needs to be addressed early in a program so that the tools are available to measure success. Models frequently can play a role in this stage, and new diagnostic tools may be needed (CDC 1993b; Gambhir et al. 2010; Hall and Fauci 2009; Marais and Pai 2007). Specificity becomes increasingly important as false positives are a huge distraction to a program in the final stages. Algorithms for diagnostic procedures need to be defined.

In the onchocerciasis elimination initiative in the Americas, the program has been challenged to meet their elimination criteria, which rely on capturing a sufficient number of black flies (the vector) to look for transmission. In some areas, the required number of flies has not been met despite extraordinary efforts. Although it is obvious that a lack of vectors is a good thing, from a disease transmission perspective, this poses a problem in terms of ensuring that elimination criteria have been met.

Another example derives from the LF initiative. To start a program, a community must demonstrate that 1% of the population is infected to initiate mass treatment. When it comes to stopping the program, they have to prove that less than 1% of people are infected. In the early protocols that were developed, this meant that 3,000 school-aged children needed to be sampled. This is a huge sample. It is programmatically very challenging, expensive, and has resulted in huge backups in the laboratory. In an effort to simplify this process, modeling based on data from well-defined populations is being used to identify new sampling protocols currently under development.

Understanding Transmission and R_0

Insufficient knowledge of transmission, and what is required to break transmission, has led to disappointment in many programs (Table 6.1). To block transmission and eliminate disease, an understanding of transmission is a basic prerequisite. For many current programs, however, understanding is insufficient, thus posing one of the greatest challenges to many ongoing initiatives today.

Leprosy is one of the oldest scourges affecting humankind, yet it is also one of the most poorly understood. Despite all of our technical advances, transmission of leprosy remains a mystery. Although the prevalence rates of leprosy have decreased—some even meet the targets of < 1 case per 10,000 population—the incidence of cases has not decreased in many areas of the world. We do not understand how or why multidrug treatment has been unable to stop transmission. This simple fact has not been embraced by the program. Consequently, there has been limited debate and insufficient research to be able to modify and expand the program beyond the current approach (Broekmans et al. 2002; Lockwood and Suneetha 2005; Vashishtha 2009). This is a major limitation and poses a threat to the program's success.

In both LF and onchocerciasis, understanding R_0 is a significant discussion point, involving a complex combination of factors (Gambhir et al. 2010) related to:

- the infection level in the community prior to the start of the control program and mass drug administration;
- the vector efficiency, density, and annual biting rate;
- the years of high-level coverage at the community level; and
- the rates of systematic noncompliance.

Modeling is helpful, but new data indicate that models need to be modified for local situations and frequently use variables that are not easily measured in the field. For onchocerciasis, we may only be able to determine R_0 after the successful elimination in the Americas, once data is collected on the vectors and indicators of infection in humans after the programs are successful and no recurrence has been observed. Even when the R_0 may be known for the Americas, the usefulness of this information in Africa remains questionable, because of the different vectors and transmission dynamics (WHO/APOC

2009). Ultimately it is this elusive figure that we would like to know and measure to prove that the job is done. Work is continuing in both the LF and onchocerciasis programs to define and refine the elimination criteria and measures of success as new data becomes available.

In Chagas disease, new transmission risks have been identified over the course of the project, causing adjustment to be made in ongoing elimination efforts. The transmission of Chagas comes from the bite of infected triatomines, primarily *Triatoma infestan*. These insects live in the walls of poor-quality huts, which are generally associated with people living in poverty. The approach to the disease has relied on improved housing, as treatment has been inadequate, particularly for the chronic stage of the disease, and good insecticides for the vector do not exist. Progress has been made in vector control, but treatment still lags; thus the focus of the program remains on improved housing. Due to transmission, the distribution of cases is almost exclusively in the rural poor parts of the Americas. However, the detection of cases in more urban centers led to the discovery of a new mechanism for transmission: one that is linked to blood transfusions. Advances in the control of the blood supply, spurred by HIV, were used to improve screening for Chagas in endemic settings. Finally, as programs have had success with these approaches, the remaining transmission mode which now dominates is congenital infection. Unfortunately, little is being done to counteract this. The current strategy involves waiting until infected women are out of their childbearing years (Dias 2009; Schmunis et al. 1996). However, attention should be given to the early detection of infected infants to facilitate treatment. In addition, recent case investigations have implicated oral transmission in some settings. Thus, the program will thus have to work to understand the implications of this on their elimination plans.

The essential lesson is that we need to follow the pattern of cases to detect new transmission patterns. As a program progresses, nondominant transmission mechanisms gain importance. Research into the mode of transmission and how to approach it early on will help a program counteract bottlenecks later.

Monitoring and Evaluation: Learning while Doing versus Formal Operational Research

The neonatal tetanus (NNT) elimination program in Egypt demonstrates the importance of using surveillance data to adapt programs and the essential element of flexibility in programming. The NNT program initiated what was felt to be an aggressive plan in 1988, based on the globally accepted approach that used annual nationwide tetanus toxoid vaccination and targeted pregnant women from 1988–1993. The campaigns were held in two rounds: one month apart in November and December each year with the participation of multiple partners, nongovernmental organizations (NGOs), and advocacy activities. Although this increased coverage immediately from 7% to 85%, and subsequently brought down NNT incidence from 3.7 per 1000 live births to 1.6 per 1000 live births, it was still above the elimination target. In looking deeper into the data, a few areas (governorates) were found to be responsible for a disproportionate number of cases: 66% of the cases were reported in areas with only 32% of the population. This led to a learning-while-doing approach, which targeted the high-incidence areas to improve routine coverage and expanded the target population of the campaign to cover all married women of childbearing age, regardless of pregnancy. Although this improved indicators, the highest risk areas still posed a problem. Thus a high-risk strategy was implemented: the governorates were subdivided into their districts, all women of childbearing age were targeted regardless of marital status, and there was significant involvement of the local communities. This was accompanied by work to improve reporting and surveillance data. With these investments as well as improved surveillance, which should increase the reporting of cases, incidence of NNT was brought for the first time down to 0.6 per 1000 live births, below the 1 per 1000 target (CDC 1996). This example illustrates the importance of data to drive programs.

The line distinguishing formal research versus dynamic programming from monitoring and learning can be blurred when a program incorporates a test-and-adapt approach. Here, a frequent weakness is the lack of in-depth monitoring as well as a lack of publication of the experience, from which other programs could learn. Planning for this type of learning should be factored into the research plan, and appropriate data should be collected to assist decision making. In addition, information should be disseminated so that programs can adopt new practices if needed.

The guinea worm eradication program in India lobbied for all program managers to be trained in basic operational research techniques to support the program. They outlined a basic framework that included considerations of the health system resources, service delivery, and the beneficiary or consumer (Kumar 1990). Empowerment of the program managers to be critical thinkers and problem solvers likely played a role in the program's success.

Case Reports

All monitoring plans should include some level of case investigation and reporting. Because reporting and intensity of investigation may increase over the lifetime of the project as cases decrease, the need to understand why a case occurs increases in a reciprocal fashion. Case investigation can be a key part of setting research priorities. Case reports have informed programs related to tuberculosis, *Haemophilus influenzae* type b (Hib), Chagas, guinea worm, and polio and have resulted in changes to the program or new research. Case reports are crucial for identifying resistance or programmatic failures (CDC 1993b; Broekmans et al. 2002; Dias 2009; Donnelly et al. 2003; Howie et al.

2007; Kumar 1990; Lemon and Robertson 1991). Case reports are also where you identify the outliers and detect the unexpected.

The Ends of the Bell Curve: When Outliers Matter

In trying to eliminate and eradicate a disease, a large proportion of the population and their communities will be addressed through minor modifications of the program. Unfortunately, in disease eradication, this is not enough. Success relies on reaching the critical proportion of the population to stop all disease transmission, and this involves not just the center of the bell curve but the outliers as well.

The current barriers within the polio program reflect the ends of the bell curve beautifully. In India, the barrier is technical: the challenge is the failure of a successfully delivered intervention. The failure is the lack of immunity conferred from the oral vaccine in Indian children from some areas. This is believed to be related to the local ecology of both the gut flora and the environment, resulting in intense exposure to intestinal pathogens early in life which alter the ability to respond effectively to the oral vaccine. In Nigeria, the problem is just the opposite: failure is due to a lack of understanding of the sociobehavioral axis of acceptance of the intervention, resulting in failure to deliver the vaccine. This difference was detected by monitoring the number of doses of vaccine given to acute flaccid paralysis and polio cases, which were identified through surveillance. In India, children have received many doses of vaccine, and the vaccine itself is not conferring immunity; in Nigeria cases have never been immunized, so the delivery system was broken. The key to overcoming both of these barriers lies in the program's ability to detect cases, understand why there are setbacks, and having a dynamic approach to address the challenges based on the underlying cause. Local site-specific problem solving and monitoring should be reviewed to set new research priorities.

The Unexpected

Expecting the unexpected may be too much to ask; however, it is important to be receptive to the unexpected so that programs can detect changes in patterns and respond. There are many examples that get even more interesting as programs approach the finish line.

In southern Mali, a poor farmer infected with guinea worm walked 400 km by foot when his fields were struck by drought. He contaminated a watering hole in an area that had never had a case of guinea worm, and this resulted in an outbreak among the nomadic warring tribes in northern Mali.

The Yanomami, who inhabit the Amazon rainforest across the border of Brazil and Venezuela, pose a challenge for the elimination of onchocerciasis in the Americas. This group is comprised of several tribes, mostly nomadic and some xenophobic, that kill any non-Yanomami on sight. This poses a challenge for community-based drug distribution. Helicopters are used for drug distribution, but migration patterns are not stable so flights have been made to a location only to find a community gone. In such a case, community engagement can help, taking advantage of local knowledge, good surveillance, good communication, case reports, and creative problem solving early on to address hard to reach populations and approaches to gain trust. New communication tools (e.g., cell phones, Twitter, Google Earth) could potentially be applied to address these issues. Operational research focused on using these tools in new initiatives would be valuable.

Empowering the Field

No one knows the field better than those who live within and are part of the culture. External observations and learning can help provide perspective and objectivity, but some of the most amazing things can happen from the field innovating for themselves. As an example, during the recent 2006 introduction of Japanese encephalitis (JE) vaccine into India, the successful introduction was thought to be impossible by most international experts with good reason: India had not introduced a new vaccine, they had never conducted an injectable vaccine campaign, there was no external financing available, the only available supply of vaccine came from China, and JE was not an international priority. JE was, however, a national and local priority. All of these barriers were overcome in an 8-month period of time to prevent further JE outbreaks triggered when a seasonal outbreak drew international attention, and the background work had been done to provide the supportive data for decision making. During this dynamic process, much innovation happened at the field level to prepare for introduction. At the national level, immunization safety and waste disposal had been discussed and debated for several years. Among the hotly debated issues were needle cutters to remove the sharp (needle) from the syringe and decrease the volume of the medical sharps waste for disposal. The JE campaigns targeted over 9 million children in their first year. There was concern over what would be done about the volume of sharp medical waste. Safety boxes were to be provided, but in the state of West Bengal they asked for needle cutters, which they were told were not available by the central level due to the ongoing debate. So, they developed their own for use in the campaigns by constructing a plastic container with a wire cutter attached (Figure 6.1). This way the needles could be disposed of as sharps, decreasing the sharps waste by over 90%. This innovation was very effective and had significant ownership at the local level.

The lesson here is twofold: What may look impossible from the global or national level may be possible when affected communities are motivated. In addition, innovations from the field can identify solutions, frequently very cost effective, that would not have otherwise been considered at central levels.

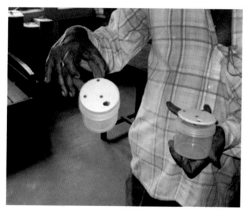

Figure 6.1   Needle cutter that was locally produced in West Bengal, India, for the Japanese encephalitis immunization campaign (picture by Julie Jacobson).

Elimination, Eradication, and the Treatment of the Patient

Technically, almost no elimination or eradication program depends on the treatment of ill or infected patients and their sequelae. The importance of a patient lies in their ability to *transmit* disease. This is evident in the focus of different programs that exclude some or all patient treatment as elements of the interventions for elimination or eradication. The following are a few examples that all represent different challenges in this paradox and the program's approach: human African trypanosomiasis (HAT), LF, and tuberculosis.

The Pan African Tsetse and Trypanosomiasis Eradication Campaign (PATTEC) approach to HAT eradication is based completely on the elimination of the vector and not the pathogen or the disease. Technically, no treatment needs to occur for this program to be successful. What does this mean from a public health perspective? Can you call it a success if you eliminate the tsetse fly while allowing all infected patients from this 100% fatal illness to die? The dynamic tension between treatment of the individual and the prevention of disease are felt most when there are limited human and financial resources with which to work. I would postulate that both need to be addressed to meet the public health needs and should therefore be included in the program for success. To complement the PATTEC approach, a screen-and-treat program with donated drugs is being conducted through separate funding by WHO and NGOs like Medicine Sans Frontiers to assist affected countries (Ahmad 2003; Kabayo 2002; Rogers and Randolph 2002).

The focus of the tuberculosis elimination initiative is treatment of smear-positive adults (Broekmans et al. 2002; CDC 1998; Vashishtha 2009). This, however, leaves other forms of tuberculosis unattended programmatically and stands in stark contrast to a clinician's duty to treat all disease and prevent suffering and death. Most programs have addressed this issue, and treatment is available for all patients clinically ill with tuberculosis regardless of the location of the pathogen, although technically it would only be necessary from the elimination perspective to treat those patients able to transmit disease. With the focus on smear-positive patients, the biggest challenge to the program is a diagnostic gap for pediatric diagnosis, detection of latent disease, and resistance. From an elimination perspective, undetected cases, latent disease, and resistance are the primary risks to ongoing transmission (CDC 1998; Dye and Williams 2008; Marais and Pai 2007). Pediatric populations present a unique challenge as they frequently have lower numbers of bacteria and do not give good sputum specimens for diagnosis, thus greatly decreasing the sensitivity of the test. This is similar to the challenge seen with the latent cases: latent disease can progress to an active state and reestablish transmission. In low-transmission countries, detecting and treating these cases based on screening of high-risk populations (e.g., immigrants from high-incidence countries, people held in institutions or prisons, and HIV-positive populations) constitute a vital component of the elimination plan (Broekmans et al. 2002; CDC 1998). In high-risk countries, these people remain mostly untreated. Diagnostic tests that can quickly detect resistance are needed to guide the appropriate selection of therapies and isolation of drug-resistant patients to stop the spread of resistance; this process is slow and cumbersome from cultured sputum specimens. All of this work depends on good surveillance data with sufficient detail to detect new trends. For example, when the association with HIV was discovered in the United States, a program began in 1993 to collect data on HIV with the newly reported tuberculosis cases (CDC 1998). This observation uncovered a new prominent driver of infection that was important to address.

Debate on this topic continues in the LF and trachoma programs, where surgery and other preventative tools are required but are frequently not funded (Perera et al. 2007). For Chagas, an approach is used that focuses on the vector, both through indoor residual spraying and improved housing in the lower resource rural areas where the disease is endemic. Interestingly, disease patterns did shift and this allowed urban transmission to be detected, which was subsequently traced back to blood transfusion. This, in turn, increased attention to the problem and initiated a program to improve the safety and screening of donated blood in affected countries. Effective treatment for patients in the chronic phase of Chagas is controversial; thus all focus is on prevention (Broekmans et al. 2002; Dias 2007, 2009). Although, in this case, there is no moral dilemma, research into new tools is needed to address the clinical pathology, prevent disease progression, and eliminate the human reservoir of infection. Even if the treatment does not eliminate disease, the treatment of patients must be considered as part of a program to increase acceptance by the community and health professionals, increase uptake of preventative measures, leverage funding to expand programs, and to relieve suffering.

Looking for Patterns

Different tools lead to different failures. For example, with a vaccine you do not have resistance; however, there are limitations in the host's ability to respond to the vaccine. This cannot be screened for by culturing pathogens and can only be followed through ongoing sensitive surveillance. Vaccines are extremely powerful tools but are frequently limited by their precision. Pneumococcal vaccine, for example, is limited since it covers only a subset of pneumococcal serotypes in the conjugated vaccine. These serotypes vary according to geographic areas and times of life. This means that the effectiveness of the pneumo vaccine depends on the pathogenic serotypes in a community and the age of the population.

The second limitation of a vaccine is the host response. No vaccine is 100% efficacious. Depending on the type of vaccine, different parts of the immune system are activated and multiple doses may be required to seroconvert or to obtain sufficient sustainable levels of antibodies and cellular immunity. Examples of limited seroconversion and inadequate immune response in polio have led to the development of monovalent vaccines to improve strain-specific immunity. The initial polio vaccine that was used as the basis for eradication is an oral vaccine, which contains the three types of polio. The trade-off for having all three types in one vaccine is having lower levels of antibodies for each and needing more doses to get an adequate immune response to all three types. This fact combined with a much deeper understanding of transmission patterns—recognizing which strains were coming from where—allows a more focused vaccine to be used to stop transmission. At the beginning of the program, knowing if an acute flaccid paralysis patient was polio positive or negative sufficed; as the program progressed, however, the need for more detailed and accurate data, including the type of polio and where the infection originated, was required.

Measles provides another example. The measles vaccine is a single dose with high seroconversion (greater than 90%). However, a second opportunity is necessary to have high enough immunity at the population level to stop transmission and outbreaks. For drugs, failure comes with increasing resistance due to selective pressure on the pathogen allowing resistant organisms to flourish, and in some cases replace, the original circulating pathogen. This can be monitored through treatment failures and culturing of the pathogen if possible (for viruses and bacteria) to determine how common these strains are and by what mechanism the resistance has developed. Early malaria eradication and tuberculosis elimination programs have confronted issues of drug resistance that have required new approaches and strategies to be developed (CDC 1993b; Hall and Fauci 2009). With both vaccine and drug approaches, monitoring the program impact is necessary to detect hypo-responsiveness and allows issues to be addressed as they arise. Part of the operational research agenda should look for such possibilities as well as what response would be required and implications for new tools that may need to be developed.

Observing programs to detect patterns can reveal synergies and new opportunities. This has led to the integration of seven of the programs for neglected tropical diseases that are now approached through an integrated platform, with community-based mass drug administration as the focal point of the programs. In addition, this has allowed the strengths of the platforms built for a specific disease, such as LF or schistosomiasis, to be utilized for seven diseases, thus expanding the scope and impact of the projects. This has been an important element in enhancing efforts for schistosomiasis, trachoma, and LF elimination. However, questions remain: Have we exploited common strategies enough? What could LF learn from the malaria experience or onchocerciasis share with efforts to eliminate HAT?

What is considered a minor part in one strategy may significantly impact another. For example, the deployment of long-lasting bed nets for malaria may have a large impact on the transmission of LF in co-endemic areas. How can we build on these opportunities? The SAFE strategy for trachoma elimination is an acronym for surgery, antibiotics, face washing, and environmental improvement. The last two points rely on provision of water and sanitation where it does not exist. When looking at the other neglected diseases, schistosomiasis and soil-transmitted helminthes could greatly benefit from water and sanitation. Could the case be made for further support by building a stronger evidence base to support these activities with additional funds as part of the plan for successful elimination and sustainability of impact? Programs will continue to struggle for funding, and this kind of integrated thinking could help us accomplish more with less by working together.

New Era of Embracing Research as Part of the Program

Currently, the best example of truly embracing research is the MalERA project, which is being developed in support of the renewed efforts to achieve malaria eradication. This call for eradication was made knowing that the necessary tools were not yet available to finish the task, but with hope that they will be in the near future and that they will be able to be introduced into programs to achieve the goal. From the beginning of the effort, this has set a tone of receptivity to new approaches and the desire to know. Hence there is regular debate and discussion on the creation of the plan for eradication, which includes a full research agenda. The MalERA project is a new community-based initiative that supports the development of a Malaria Eradication Research Agenda (MalERA) (Hall and Fauci 2009). The project encourages participation from the broader malaria community as well as creative, critical, and innovative thinking and is addressing the full spectrum of tools, strategies, and implementation. Thus far seven themes have been identified and are currently being explored through scientific and technical workshops, dialog with lead research agencies, and solicited input through the internet including: drugs, vaccines, vector control, modeling, monitoring/evaluation/surveillance, integration strategies, and health systems/operations. The key considerations and research approaches are summarized in the case study below. This project is to be praised not only for its inclusive process but also for the publication of the research agenda in several formats for comment and debate.

For successful malaria eradication, the essential goal of the strategy is to stop transmission and break the parasite life cycle. The challenges are many and focus around the complex life cycle of the pathogen and the diversity of settings in which malaria is transmitted as well as the adaptability of the parasite and the vector, interactions with the human host and the control program. The current strategy for control is combined drug therapy to treat patients and combat resistance, vector control with indoor residual spraying and insecticide-treated bed nets to prevent transmission, and strategies to identify and treat cases early. Social, economic, and behavioral factors all influence the human interaction with the parasite life cycle. Challenges in this area relate to compliance with prevention efforts and treatment as well as willingness to buy only combination therapy to decrease the emergence of resistance. In areas where interventions are currently successful and disease levels fall, two types of new challenges arise: (a) programmatic and political, keeping attention on sustaining the efforts and the investment for control, and (b) technical, detection and accurate diagnosis of cases as prevalence decreases. This demonstrates the importance of approaching problems and issues from both a programmatic perspective as well as a biomedical perspective. To stop transmission, the strategy will need to expand from treatment of sick patients to include detection and treatment of asymptomatic cases that can sustain transmission. This will require new and different diagnostics with the ability to have appropriate sensitivity and specificity with lower population prevalence and parasite density.

To move the malaria research and development effort forward, the National Institute of Allergy and Infectious Diseases (NIAID) is playing a central role and has committed to the pursuit of the following goals (NIAID and NIH 2008a):

1. Increase fundamental understanding of the complex interactions among malaria parasites, the mosquito vectors responsible for their transmission, and the human host.
2. Strengthen the ability to identify, develop, validate, and evaluate new tools and strategies for treatment, prevention, and control of malaria.
3. Enhance both national and international research and the research training infrastructure to meet malaria research needs, particularly for community-based and community-supported clinical trials in malaria endemic countries.

4. Advance research to develop tools to support and sustain global efforts to control, eliminate, and eventually eradicate malaria.

In the research agenda, work is ongoing to identify weak spots in the life cycle or ecology of transmission. The life cycle of the parasite has key biological bottlenecks that are the focus of interventions: the initial point of infection, when there are few parasites and uptake of the sexual stage of the parasite by the mosquito. Research is now focused on taking advantage of these weak points. *Plasmodium falciparum* has dominated the thinking in malaria globally due to severity of disease and resistance. If malaria eradication is to be successful, all malaria parasites will need to be addressed. Each parasite presents a different challenge and will require a different research investment (Hall and Fauci 2009; NIAID and NIH 2008a, b).

The discussion and plan to address these issues is ongoing. Table 6.2 shows some of the research needs identified. Only time will tell how effective these efforts are and how this research will support and guide the program. However, they provide a new paradigm for embracing research as a part of an eradication program.

From the work done on malaria we can devise some generalizations and reflections for other diseases:

- Focus on the weak points in transmission that could be the focal points for interventions.
- Social and behavioral issues at the individual, community and global level need to be studied and interventions found.
- Inclusive proactive process, from the beginning of the project, can establish a culture that is receptive to change.
- Innate epidemiology will shift as the program progresses, and assumptions will need to be retested as transmission dynamics change.
- Tool requirements will vary at different stages of a program and thus need to be thought about early to be ready in time.

Yin and Yang

Elimination and eradication efforts are an optimist's sport. If you are not an optimist, the reasons why any program can or will fail can be overwhelming. However, unbridled or ignorant optimism constitutes an important reason why programs fail. Keys to success are critical thinking, innovative problem solving, persistence, and high levels of energy. To encourage critical thinking and problem solving, a program should invite the critics to the table and the pessimists into the debate. They can help point out weaknesses in the program and potential barriers to success that can help to guide the research agenda.

Developing the Research Plan

Research is an essential component to an elimination or eradication program. In developing a research strategy in support of a program, it is important to learn from our history as demonstrated above. One approach is to look at the criteria that determined that the pathogen was able to be eliminated (Table 6.3) (Molyneux et al. 2004) and determine how to monitor these characteristics, where the weak spots are in the plan and what backup strategies would need to be developed.

Look at all areas of potential failure: the tool, the delivery system, the strategy, and detection and response to the unexpected. This framework can be used to design the crucial elements of the research plan (Figure 6.2). The research agenda should consider how it responds to new data from monitoring and evaluation programs as well as how new data generated through research is used to guide programming. Early deliberation should define what success would look like and how it would be measured. Criteria to start programs are frequently easier and more straightforward than criteria to stop an intervention. Thus, early attention should be paid to stopping criteria and the additional tools that may be required. The plan should allow for innovation from the field and early communication, discussion, and dissemination of results.

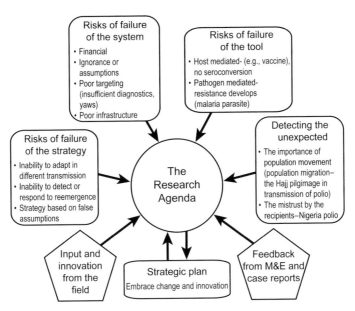

Figure 6.2   Framework for establishing research priorities in elimination or eradication programs. M&E: monitoring and evaluation.

Table 6.2 Epidemiologic states and examples of priority research requirements.

Status:	Epidemiologic features:	Priority research requirements:
Current situation	1.3 M deaths/yr (mostly children)	Expand research on non-falciparum malaria
	300–500 M clinical cases/yr	Expand research on combination drug therapy
	Children and young pregnant women are primary at-risk populations	Expand research and development for malaria vaccines
	4–5 species infecting humans, including *Plasmodium falciparum, P. vivax,* and *P. knowlesi*	Expand research on vector biology and ecology on non-gambiae Anopheline mosquitoes
	Some areas with very high entomological inoculation rates (EIRs)	
1. Control*	Widespread drug resistance	Assure and expand pipeline of available interventions (drugs, vaccines, insecticides/repellents, diagnostics)
	Ongoing surveillance documents:	Assess degree of parasite population diversity to discover, identify, validate, evaluate, and optimize interventional tools and strategies
	Decrease incidence and prevalence of disease in areas where control has been implemented	Develop mathematical models based on emerging field data to help guide product development and optimize combinations of interventions
2. Elimination of disease*	Ongoing surveillance documents:	Assess changing epidemiology of malaria, including shifts in burden of disease and source of gametocytes
	No deaths directly attributed to malaria	Adapt tools and interventions to situation of decreasing incidence and prevalence
	Incidence and prevalence of uncomplicated malaria is falling and/or low	
	EIRs can still sustain infection	

Table 6.2 (continued)

Status	Epidemiologic features:	Priority research requirements:
3. Elimination of infection*	Ongoing surveillance documents:	Assess changing epidemiology of malaria, including shifts in burden of disease and source of gametocytes
	No deaths directly attributed to malaria	
	Low and falling prevalence of parasitemia	Adapt tools and interventions to situation of low incidence and prevalence (e.g., improved diagnostics for surveillance in mosquito populations)
	Low incidence, mainly due to short epidemics that are rapidly identified, treated, and contained	Evaluate utility of transmission reduction strategies (e.g., transmission-blocking vaccines, transgenic mosquitoes)
	Low EIRs, whether due to low rates of infection in mosquitoes, decreased vectorial capacity or reduced biting behavior	
	Drug and insecticide resistance is identified prospectively and managed	
4. Eradication*	No malaria deaths	Develop validated, rapid, highly sensitive diagnostics for detection of human and mosquito infections during surveillance period
	Prevalence = 0	
	Incidence = 0	
	EIR = 0	

*According to International Task Force on Disease Eradication in order of progression (earlier to later).

Table 6.3 Criteria for targeting a disease for eradication and the subsequent research and program needs.

Biological and technical feasibility:	Research questions and program considerations:
Natural history of biological agent	Understand transmission including latent and subclinical infection, duration of pathogen in the environment
Non-human reservoirs	Define reservoirs both human and nonhuman, risks of exposure, and transmission from the reservoir
Effective intervention tool	Follow efficacy, cure, and relapse rate Detect resistance early
Effective delivery strategy	Differentiate resistance from poor delivery Define appropriate programmatic monitors that are relevant to modify the program
Simple and practical diagnostic	Can you detect latent or subclinical cases? Will you be able to detect recurrence versus reinfection? How will sensitivity vs. specificity needs of the diagnostic tool adapt as prevalence changes? What additional tests or algorithms will be needed?
Sensitive surveillance	Can you detect cases early? Where will cases present? Who will need to be sensitized to identify cases? Could cases be confused with something else? If so, what? Who are providers in the community (public, private, traditional) that will need to be included in surveillance and treatment protocols? How will you encourage reporting?
Field-proven strategies	How will strategies need to be modified in different settings? How will you detect failure of the system?

Table 6.3 (continued)

Costs and benefits:	Research questions and program considerations:
Cases averted per year	How will you measure and how often?
Coincident benefits	
Intangible benefits	How will this data be used?
Estimated annual direct global savings	How will it be presented and in what format to influence decision making at what level?
Estimated total external financing	How will you fund collection of this data?
Societal and political considerations:	Research questions and program considerations:
Political commitment (endemic and/or industrialized)	What is the measure and how will you follow?
Social support (endemic and/or industrialized)	What action will be taken if indicators shift?
Disease burden in politically unstable areas	How will you address delivery in unstable settings? Identify the different partners working in this setting.
Core partnerships and advocates	How will this be organized and monitored for effectiveness? Define roles?
Technical consensus	How will new data be discussed and deliberated? How will program/strategy updates be incorporated?
Donor base (number of donors 1M or more)	How will new donors be brought on board? How will historic donors be kept invested? How will new funding needs be met when new challenges arise? How will research and advocacy be funded?

Funding Programs and Research

In all assessments of all programs, the issue of funding will be brought up as one of the reasons for setbacks and failure. Elimination programs are greatly aided by support through selected institutions and foundations. The Nippon Foundation, for example, made a generous donation and supported the world-wide costs of leprosy elimination between 1994 and 1999, which treated more that 13 million people (Lockwood and Suneetha 2005). Rotary International and their network continue to provide significant support to the polio efforts. Lions Club has provided important funding for the Onchocerciasis Elimination Program in the Americas (OEPA). Drug donation programs for LF and oncho-cerciasis have been the cornerstone for elimination efforts. Ensuring funding sufficient to achieve the final goal is always a challenge. Providing supportive data on cost-effectiveness or cost-benefit can help programs generate program funds; however, research needs are not usually addressed through such analy-ses. Establishing the case for how research can support a program and result in cost or time savings in the long run would help in defining the value and get-ting the funds to support research. Flexibility in funding also helps a program be responsive to challenges as they arrive and is essential for elimination or eradication.

Conclusion: Guiding Principles for Research

- Criteria that establish whether a disease is able to be eliminated or eradicated can also guide the research agenda.
- Know that program targets and strategies will change over the life-time of a program and be prepared to provide the data necessary to inform the decision-making process and enable mechanisms for mod-ifying the strategy.
- Include adaptive programming with appropriate monitoring and eval-uation as part of the research agenda.
- Think through the stages of the program and the tools that will be required to anticipate needs so they don't become barriers.
- Pay attention to the ends of the Bell curve. Outliers matter in elimina-tion and eradication programs. Case reports and investigations should feed into research needs.
- The research agenda should be proactive, interactive, and incorporate innovation from the outside as well as from the bottom up, with a critical eye focused on the success of the program.
- Sufficient and flexible funding is required to address program barriers and the research agenda to support decision making.

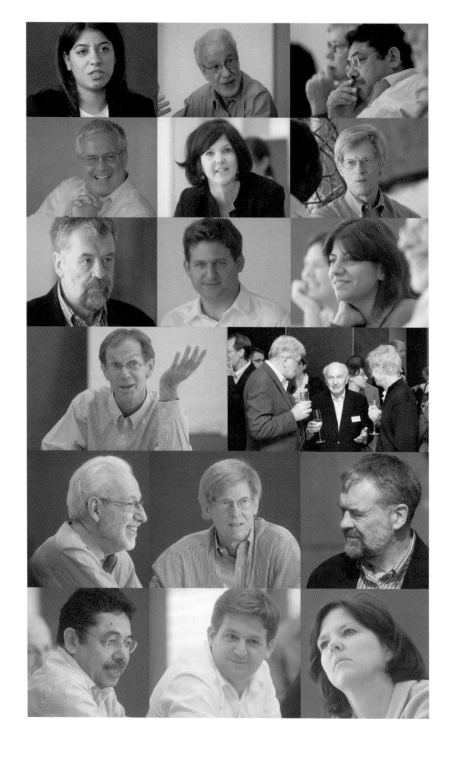

7

Group Report: Assessing the Feasibility of an Eradication Initiative

Peter Strebel, Eric A. Ottesen, Ciro A. de Quadros,
Sherine Guirguis, Robert G. Hall, Linda Muller,
Jai Prakash Narain, and Ole Wichmann

Abstract

New global eradication initiatives in the 21st century will face more stringent and rigorous pre-launch review than their predecessors. The assessment of whether a disease can and should be targeted for eradication will involve determination of whether the disease agent meets fundamental biological and technical criteria, demonstration of operational feasibility in large and/or challenging settings, and a comprehensive review of a number of critical enabling factors required for eradication.

This chapter builds on earlier work that describes the biological and technical requirements for disease eradication and focuses in more detail on nonbiological, critical enabling factors. These include durable financing, effective communication strategies, and operational research, each of which plays a cross-cutting role in building and sustaining the necessary political and societal support for eradication. An eradication investment case, program governance, and the interface with health systems are additional enabling factors that are covered in more detail in separate chapters.

Before launching a new eradication initiative, a comprehensive review of feasibility is required. If judged feasible, individual champions and a broad-based partnership will be needed to raise the political and financial support required to launch the initiative. The assessment of feasibility is not a "one-off" activity but rather needs continual monitoring and updating as new technologies and information become available.

Introduction

The criteria needed to determine whether eradication is able to be achieved have been grouped into three categories: biological, societal/political, and economic factors (Hinman and Hopkins 1998). An additional factor was emphasized by the Global Taskforce on Disease Eradication; namely, the need to demonstrate that eradication could be achieved in a large geographical area (CDC 1993b). A more recent review of lessons learned from eradication initiatives stresses that biological feasibility is necessary but not sufficient. Nonbiological factors such as political commitment, social acceptability, financial affordability, and strong program management are critical components for success (Aylward et al. 2000a).

Over the last two decades, a wealth of practical experience has been gained from global and regional eradication initiatives that have targeted diseases such as polio, guinea worm, lymphatic filariasis, onchocerciasis, measles, and rubella. The global context in which eradication programs operate has, however, markedly changed during this time. Sudden events, such as high-profile terrorist attacks, large-scale natural disasters, and the 2008 financial crisis, as well as secular trends in the size and age structure of the world's population and the continuing shift from rural to metropolitan areas, globalization, the decentralization and privatization of health services, and increased connectivity through information technology have changed the landscape dramatically. Support for disease eradication programs has also significantly changed: at ever-increasing rates, highly influential nongovernmental organizations and foundations are now involved, and there has been a corresponding decline in the technical, operational, and financial monopoly previously held by multilateral international organizations such as the World Health Organization, UNICEF, and the World Bank.

Over the past decade, the rise in corporate social responsibility has led to an increased involvement of corporations in global public health initiatives. Commensurate with this has been the drive to create innovative financing mechanisms and apply business models and management principles to public health programs. In addition, communication technology has changed considerably. The burgeoning use of social media and the Internet have altered how individuals and communities are able to impact policymaking on health issues and acceptance of the interventions required for eradication. Any side effects from these interventions (e.g., adverse events following vaccination) can quickly achieve prominence on the political and media agendas.

Understanding the complex interaction between disease agents and the interventions used in an eradication initiative is crucial. The need to continue control measures indefinitely—albeit of a different kind and on a smaller scale—has increasingly been recognized. In addition, should eradication be achieved, surveillance at some level is necessary and control of laboratory activities involving pathogens must be maintained (e.g., laboratory containment of polioviruses and management of the remaining stocks of smallpox virus).

In view of these developments, our group was tasked with assessing the feasibility of achieving an eradication goal in the 21st century. Building on earlier work (Dowdle and Hopkins 1998; CDC 1993b), we address the cross-cutting role of sustainable financing, effective communication strategies, and operational research in building the necessary political and societal support for eradication. We include discussion of additional critical enabling factors (e.g., an investment case, program governance, and an effective interface with health systems) and conclude with a set of conclusions and recommendations.

Assessing the Feasibility of Eradication

We expect that disease eradication initiatives in the 21st century will face more stringent and rigorous pre-launch review than their predecessors. The assessment of whether a disease can and should be targeted for eradication will involve three primary stages: (a) determination of whether the disease agent meets fundamental feasibility criteria, (b) demonstration of operational feasibility in large and/or challenging settings, and (c) a comprehensive review of a number of critical enabling factors required for eradication.

Fundamental Feasibility Criteria

The distinct biological attributes of an organism and the performance characteristics of interventions determine the potential for eradication. These biological and technical criteria have been discussed and reported on in detail (Ottesen et al. 1998) and are therefore summarized below.

Biological Feasibility

Biological feasibility depends on the inherent properties of the agent and the disease it causes. When humans are essential for the life cycle of the agent, eradication is most feasible, because it is possible to apply an effective intervention tool to humans and interrupt transmission of the agent (Ottesen et al. 1998). This certainly was the case for smallpox eradication. The successful eradication of rinderpest, a disease of cattle and domestic buffalo, expands this concept to include a reservoir for infection in humans or other easily identifiable species. A restricted reservoir enables problems to be quickly identified and targeted interventions to be effectively applied. Other attributes of the agent may also impact eradicability: transmission potential, susceptibility to reinfection, duration of infectiousness and recrudescence, and persistence of the agent in the environment.

Technical Feasibility

To achieve eradication, an effective intervention (e.g., a vaccine or medication) to stop transmission and practical, accurate diagnostic tools to determine who is infected are necessary. Vaccines, therapeutic agents, behavior modification, vector control, or a combination thereof must be of sufficient efficacy to interrupt transmission of the agent. Similarly, diagnostic tools must have sufficient sensitivity and specificity to detect infection and be relatively simple to use in diverse settings. The concept of what constitutes an effective intervention or accurate diagnostic tools, however, changes over time as the result of scientific advancement and technical innovations.

Demonstration of Operational Feasibility

The availability of an effective intervention at the individual level does not mean that an automatic scale-up is possible at the population level. Demonstration that eradication can be achieved in a large geographic area provides proof of this principle. In addition, the experience from the polio eradication initiative indicates that interventions need to be tested and tailored (e.g., monovalent and bivalent oral polio vaccine) before they can effectively meet the most challenging settings (e.g., where routine immunization coverage is the lowest and the herd immunity threshold is the highest). Operational feasibility must be viewed as an ongoing process. During the course of an eradication initiative, novel challenges may emerge for which there are no pat solutions. Thus, the criteria necessary for operational feasibility must be considered separately from the more fundamental biological and technical criteria.

In addition to being effective, an ideal intervention needs to be safe, cheap, and easy to apply. This will increase acceptance by communities and support early adoption into national programs. Research should be conducted throughout the course of an eradication program to ensure that "field-friendly" interventions and tools with improved product profiles are developed.

Critical Enabling Factors

Because of their nonbiological nature, critical enabling factors are generally more amenable to organizational and managerial interventions. Understanding the process for developing and maintaining political and societal support is crucial to the success of an eradication effort. Before embarking on new eradication initiatives, a comprehensive assessment of the following enabling factors is required.

Political Commitment

Success of eradication initiatives is dependent on a consistently high level of political support and engagement far beyond that engendered by national Ministries of Health. Commitment is needed from Heads of State, national parliaments, as well as from provincial and district governments as well as traditional and local community leaders. Before starting an eradication initiative, it is imperative to build the necessary political support at country, regional, and global levels. Depending on the nature of the interventions required for eradication, intersectoral collaboration across different governmental departments may be required (e.g., support from the education department is crucial for vaccination campaigns in schools). Political commitment, in turn, has to be translated into financial allocations at the country level. Coordination of the various parties is crucial. For example, during polio eradication activities, Interagency Coordinating Committees played a key role in bringing together in-country partners (NGOs, bilateral agencies, international organizations, and the private sector) and government representatives to ensure that the program was fully funded.

A combination of incentives and disincentives is needed to leverage full country participation at the global level and full stakeholder participation within each country. In the polio experience, for example, a World Health Assembly resolution, while nonbinding, served as a useful instrument to exert political pressure on a country to improve performance. Eradication programs in the 21st century may, however, require additional mechanisms (e.g., binding agreements or treaties) to secure formal commitment from governments and partners and to maintain this commitment when setbacks occur.

At the country and community level, lessons from the polio program clearly show that when traditional and religious leaders are engaged as champions and stewards of eradication programs, community acceptance and coverage of immunization campaigns increases. In the Americas, the experience gained from the polio, measles, and rubella initiatives highlights the importance of engaging professional medical societies (e.g., pediatricians, obstetricians, and gynecologists) as well as private sector hospitals and clinics to enhance advocacy, communication, and disease surveillance. Surveys of policy makers may be useful in identifying key stakeholders and potential barriers to success as well as in assessing what actions or information are needed to maximize political commitment (DeRoeck 2004).

Societal Support

While earlier eradication programs may have relied on the personal experience and intuition of program managers to engage with communities, new eradication initiatives face more informed and potentially more assertive communities. Thus, an eradication program will benefit from applying a structured approach to engage effectively with the community and establish trust.

Behavior change theories and field experience have shown that communities support health initiatives when they perceive that a disease is severe and has the potential to harm them or their families. In turn, they will demand access to the intervention being provided if they believe it to be a safe, effective, and an accessible response to their health needs.

Generating demand for a health service first involves identifying key community stakeholders with whom to engage and target for supporting an intervention. It is important to understand the reasons why these stakeholders may support or resist the intervention being offered (this kind of analysis should be done based on a communication theory model). Next, potential strategies for overcoming social barriers or exploiting existing opportunities should be tested and implemented in the field. Field experience from the polio program has demonstrated that the messenger is equally, if not more, critical at times than the message itself; thus targeted messages should be delivered by influential champions who carry credibility and trust. Societal support for an eradication program should be continuously monitored through knowledge, attitudes, and practices surveys and other social research. Health staff (e.g., at community health centers and clinics) play a key role in engaging with local communities and serve as critical brokers between the eradication program and the local community. To sustain their commitment and to enable them to garner community support for the duration required in an eradication program, health staff are likely to require continuous training, support, and motivation to persevere as the critical foot soldiers in an eradication program.

Strong Economic and Ethical Arguments

To build the required financial support for an eradication program, an investment case or business plan is necessary—one that addresses the expected costs and benefits of an eradication program as well as delivers an approach to manage risks and provides an exit strategy (see Thompson et al., this volume). The investment case must include an independent assessment of how a specific proposed eradication initiative meets the feasibility criteria discussed above as well as the critical enabling factors identified in this section. Emerson (this volume) proposes that the moral case for eradication should be based on arguments such as the duty to rescue, duty to future generations, societal health equity, and disease eradication as a global public good.

Demonstration of Financial Feasibility

As a result of the 2008 financial crisis, competition for the funding of global public health and eradication programs has intensified. Future disease eradication initiatives will thus need to include a financial feasibility study as a core component of the eradication decision-making process. Such a financial feasibility study must assess the projected financial costs (and possible range of costs), the likelihood of the required funds being made available, and the fiscal attributes of the funds (e.g., their ability to be front-loaded, flexible, predictable, and coordinated). The assessment of financial feasibility should estimate the proportion of funds that can be expected to come from different funding sources (e.g., national governments, partner agencies, partner governments, private sector) and the resulting implications. This includes how funds might be predicted to be earmarked (e.g., geographically and by program component, such as supplies, disease surveillance, operations, and research).

The need for global cooperation to obtain the public good of disease eradication gives credence to a "fair share" financing concept for public sector partners and could have individual countries providing financing in proportion to, for example, their assessed contribution to the WHO or their gross national income. Consideration must be given on how to manage "free-riders" (i.e., those who extract benefit from the provision of the public good without paying their "fair share"). The potential use of newer financing approaches—transaction tax mechanisms, global or regional development bank "buy-downs," bond issuance to secure up-front financing, and performance-based funding—should be explored. A financing strategy that ensures a diversity of funding sources would help protect against the risks posed by any individual funder exiting the program. An optimal financing model would also include mechanisms to monitor and evaluate financing flows and processes for addressing any deficiencies.

Effective Communication Strategies

Lessons learned from polio and other eradication programs highlight the importance of strategic communications planning as an integral component of any eradication initiative. According to Bates et al. (this volume), over the last few years developments and innovations in the field of communications have enabled communications to be applied to eradication programs through an evidence-based, systematic, and evaluable approach. Well-conceived, professionally implemented communication strategies that are directly linked to an eradication program's objectives, and which bring an understanding of political, social, and cultural realities, can make the difference between the success and failure of a program.

A framework for effective communication strategies should include at least the following principles:

- Communication is a planned process. An initial assessment should be conducted to identify all potential stakeholders, so that tailored messages and engagement strategies can be constructed for each group. Stakeholders may include politicians, professional groups, local and international partners, program staff and managers, the media, as well as the general public, including marginalized communities.
- Plan in advance for nonparticipating players. Eradication requires near-universal participation. Hence, special attention is needed to engage and reach "nonparticipating players." Experiences from other eradication initiatives indicate that those most unlikely to participate are politically or socially excluded groups, as well as inaccessible populations. While it may be unlikely that all nonparticipating players can be identified in advance, a risk assessment can be conducted to plan for most.
- Initial assumptions on knowledge, attitudes, and behaviors should be identified and tested based on a model. A communication theory model

that makes assumptions of behavioral motivation for each key social group or stakeholder should be established and continuously tested throughout the life cycle of the eradication program.

- Repeated messages through diverse communication tools are most effective. A mix of communication mechanisms and approaches is required to respond to the various factors (e.g., threat perception, self-efficacy, intervention efficacy) that are critical for behavior and attitude changes. Mass media, social mobilization, and interpersonal communication are all proven tools for communicating messages to various target groups. Expanded access to the Internet and the use of social media (e.g., blog sites, chat rooms, Facebook) provide additional communication opportunities. However, social media is also capable of rapidly spreading misinformation. Therefore, both the advantages and disadvantages of these communication tools must be carefully factored into an effective communication strategy.

- Community engagement is a central principle for all stakeholders. An exchange of information and ongoing dialog between program staff and stakeholders is necessary to foster an environment of inclusive participation and ownership among as many stakeholders as possible. The media needs to be considered as a critical stakeholder for engagement. Lavery et al. (2010) provide useful guidelines to secure engagement at the community level. Experience from both low-resource and industrialized countries has shown that as disease burden declines, societal demand declines and people become more vulnerable to reports of side effects of the intervention. To offset this, effective communication strategies are needed throughout the entire course of an eradication initiative. In addition, lessons learned in how to exact effective community engagement should be shared between the different eradication initiatives. Compiling this experience will promote a more evidence-based approach in the future.

Governance

The increasing role of private funding from corporations, foundations, and individuals has led to more stringent requirements for financial accountability, strong management, and independent monitoring of eradication initiatives. Stoever et al. (this volume) recommend that the governance structure of future eradication programs needs to be planned and structured to ensure principles of effective management, transparent accounting, and independent oversight.

Impact on Health Systems

As previously emphasized (Cochi et al. 1998), eradication programs should be planned and carried out in the context of health services; they should contribute to the strengthening of infrastructure and management weaknesses; those health systems which are least developed will need the most infrastructure support; and a functional approach should be taken to balance global, national, and local priorities. Pate et al. (this volume) provide a comprehensive discussion on how an eradication program can be designed to interface effectively with the health system. They also provide a framework for optimal engagement of disease eradication initiatives with health systems.

Operational Research Agenda

Historically, operational research efforts have been both minimally supported and insufficiently incorporated in all global eradication initiatives. The Dahlem meeting clearly identified the need for a research capacity, citing important lessons from past eradication initiatives, which clearly show that technical problems will arise and can only be resolved by operational research (Hinman and Hopkins 1998). Examples include research to develop cheaper, more effective, or easier to use interventions; field studies to improve our understanding of the epidemiology of the disease and the impact of interventions at the population level; and knowledge, attitudes, and practices surveys to guide communication strategies.

Jacobson (this volume) describes a framework that can be used to design the crucial elements of the research plan. Each criterion used to determine the feasibility of an eradication initiative needs to be tested and evaluated to determine weak spots and devise solutions. Operational research should look at all areas of potential failure: the pathogen, the intervention tools, the delivery system, communication strategies, financing, program management, as well as the detection and response to the unexpected. A research agenda must consider how it can respond to new data received from monitoring and evaluation programs as well as how new data generated through research can be used to guide programming.

To establish this program component, two principal challenges must be addressed. First, an appropriate budget should be established for operational research, with perhaps a fixed proportion of the program budget set aside for operational research (e.g., 5% or some other proportion). We note, however, that it is often very difficult for resource-constrained programs to carve from their limited implementation funds the resources required to address questions that might take years to answer. Second, a mechanism is required to ensure that when such funding exists, a fast, efficient, and coherent process is available to identify critical program challenges in need of operational research. This involves developing appropriate research protocols and advancing them to the funding sources.

A particularly good model to meet the programmatic needs for operational research appears to be the recently created Polio Research Committee of the

Global Polio Eradication Initiative. The attributes that make this model particularly strong are:

- Its very close association to and management by the program.
- Its membership is largely external but very knowledgeable about the program.
- Regular meetings are conducted, which allows for a rapid intake of proposals as problems arise.
- Its ability to support a range of projects, including those that originate in the field, those that pertain to program monitoring and end-game strategies, as well as those targeting vaccine development and further "upstream" challenges.

Further details on how the research needs of eradication initiatives can best be defined, articulated, and met are discussed by Jacobson (this volume).

What Is the Process for Establishing a New Eradication Initiative?

The Dahlem meeting (Goodman et al. 1998b) explored three different options for investigating, proposing, and selecting candidate diseases for eradication:

1. Continuation of the status quo in which diverse pathways lead to a resolution by the World Health Assembly.
2. Establishment of a unit at WHO to analyze, evaluate, and make commitments to eradicate specific diseases.
3. Establishment of an interagency work group.

The process for establishing a new global eradication initiative in the 21st century will likely require a sequential approach and may include aspects of one or more of these options. The premise holds that the role of the WHO and a World Health Assembly resolution are necessary, but not sufficient.

A number of different candidate diseases could be periodically assessed by technical advisory groups. If the biological and technical feasibility criteria are met and rapid progress is being made with accelerated control efforts, then the disease-specific partnership could advance an investment case to stakeholders and begin the process of assessing the feasibility of attaining the platform of support required to launch the eradication initiative. Once a comprehensive review of all the critical enabling factors has been conducted and results are favorable, the next step would be to initiate a resolution to establish a new global eradication goal. This would likely be brought to the World Health Assembly by a Member State(s), the WHO Secretariat, or another interested party. This process could start in the different Regional Committees of WHO, thereby ensuring full political support by all countries and regions. This approach is similar to that proposed by Foege (1998) and is illustrated in the Figure 7.1.

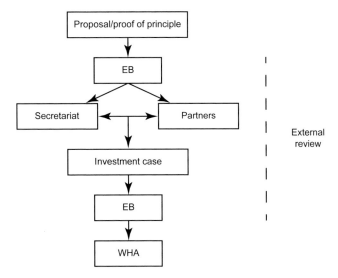

Figure 7.1 Pathway to the establishment of a World Health Assembly (WHA) resolution on disease eradication. EB: executive board.

Conclusions and Recommendations

The global context in which new disease eradication initiatives will be evaluated is rapidly evolving. The competition for public health resources requires a comprehensive review of all aspects of the feasibility of a new initiative:

1. Assessing the feasibility of a disease eradication initiative requires (a) determination of whether the disease agent and interventions meet fundamental biological and technical criteria; (b) demonstration of operational feasibility in large and/or challenging settings; and (c) a thorough review of critical enabling factors.

2. The critical enabling factors to be assessed include political commitment, societal support, strong economic and ethical arguments (as part of an eradication investment case), demonstration of financial feasibility, an effective governance structure, and the ability to positively impact health systems.

3. Effective communication strategies, operational research, and sustainable financing play an essential cross-cutting role in building the necessary political and societal support.

4. Having assessed an eradication initiative as feasible, individual champions and a broad-based partnership are needed to raise the political and financial support necessary to launch the initiative.

5. The assessment of feasibility is not a one-off activity but rather requires continual monitoring and updating as new technologies and information become available.

6. The process of establishing a new eradication initiative will likely be sequential. Once biological and technical feasibility criteria are met and rapid progress is being made with accelerated control efforts, the disease-specific partnership would then advance an eradication investment case to stakeholders.

7. The role of the WHO and a World Health Assembly resolution are necessary but not sufficient to establish a new global eradication initiative. A robust political and financial platform of support is required to successfully launch the initiative.

Issues in the Development of an Eradication Investment Case

8

The Moral Case for Eradication

Claudia I. Emerson

…it's clear that though eradication rests firmly on both chemistry
and entomology, it depends even more heavily on human beings.
—C. A. Needham and R. Canning (2003:22)

Abstract

This chapter considers the question of whether there is a moral imperative to pursue
disease eradication once we have the means to achieve it. It examines three arguments
that support the case for eradication from an ethical perspective: (a) the duty to rescue,
(b) the duty to future generations, and (c) the notion of disease eradication as a global
public good. It concludes that where disease eradication is possible, ethical motivation offers compelling reasons to act that cannot be dismissed without incurring moral
liability. Ethical considerations should thus be weighed in the balance of reasons that
inform decisions about whether or not to pursue disease eradication.

Introduction

The eradication of smallpox, hailed as one of the greatest achievements in the
history of medicine, continues to inspire efforts to eradicate other diseases that
cause immense human suffering and death. It is a testament to the evocative
power of eradication that campaigns to eradicate diseases (e.g., polio) persevere despite the many challenges that must be overcome. The challenges are
complex: scientific, technical, economic, political and sociocultural. Within
the sociocultural strand, we can locate the ethical considerations that relate to
disease eradication efforts.

Some of these considerations reflect ethical issues that arise in the context of
mass immunization programs, such as risk and benefit, adequacy of informed
consent, the tension between individual and collective interests, transparency,
and questions of resource allocation (Verweiji and Dawson 2004; Dawson
2009; Ulmer and Liu 2002; Paul 2005; Paul and Dawson 2005). Analyses
of these issues have been presented by others and those arguments will not
be repeated here. Instead, this chapter will reflect on the broader question of

whether there is an ethical imperative to pursue disease eradication once we have the means to achieve it.

If there is an obligation to pursue disease eradication, on what grounds can it be justified? The aim of this chapter is to present ethical arguments that support the case for eradication.[1] It is not claimed that ethical arguments alone make a case for eradication—ethical grounds are necessary, but insufficient. The goal is to examine ethical considerations that are compelling enough to warrant inclusion in the decision-making process. Elsewhere the ethical case for completing polio eradication has been considered (Emerson and Singer 2010), which alongside sustained analyses of the economic and scientific feasibility (Thompson and Duintjer Tebbens 2007; Barrett 2004) make the case for eradicating polio. Those arguments shall be considered in greater depth and extended to the investment case for disease eradication more generally. In many ways, polio is a paradigm case from which insights can be drawn: it is an eradicable disease that has proved elusive to eradication. It is against the backdrop of prospective eradication with its inherent technical, economic, and sociopolitical challenges that the analysis is situated.[2] Obligations to rescue and to future generations, as well as the notion of disease eradication as a global public good are examined from an ethical perspective. The conclusion is that where disease eradication is possible, ethical motivation offers compelling reasons to act that cannot be dismissed without incurring moral liability. The implication is that ethical considerations should be weighed in the balance of reasons that inform decisions about whether or not to pursue disease eradication.

Why Are Ethical Arguments Needed?

Disease has been called the true serial killer of human history, having affected more human lives than war, famine, and natural disaster (Dobson 2007). Few would readily contest that eradicating disease to save countless lives from disability and death is the right thing to do if achievable, and if doing so would not have detrimental effects on other goods on balance. Why, then, would ethical arguments in support of disease eradication be required? Articulating the ethical arguments that support eradication serves several purposes.

---

[1]   Disease eradication is not referred to here as a general strategy, but rather those instances where eradication is an appropriate strategy for a specific disease, where all of the criteria for the disease to be deemed eradicable have been met. Moreover, the question is concerned with choosing eradication over control efforts, not with choosing between different potential targets of eradication. This latter question is complex and merits its own analysis and justification within an eradication investment case.

[2]   Although the analysis is limited to eradication, some of the arguments could well apply to the case of elimination.

activities can be and are used by many developing countries as a springboard to address other health priorities" (Sutter and Cochi 1997). The cost-effectiveness of eradication is exemplified in the case of smallpox, with the United States recouping its total investment of USD 32 million every 26 days, and economic modeling showing that in the long-term eradication as a strategy offers lower cumulative costs (Thompson and Duintjer Tebbens 2007). While it is now believed that eradication does not imply the cessation of all preventive measures, an economic analysis of the GPEI clearly demonstrates that the net benefits of eradication far outweigh the rising costs to achieve it (Duintjer Tebbens et al. 2011). In addition, even with the costs of indefinitely maintaining some preventive measures, countries benefit from the substantial savings of no longer having to mount responses to outbreaks and importations. From an ethical perspective, the eradication of disease represents a tremendous investment in reducing the "human cost" of disease, which has both an economic and moral tally. This is the immeasurable cost of suffering and social disruption, of lives altered, and lives lost. It is difficult to place an economic value on what Thompson and Duintjer Tebbens (2007) refer to as "the large, intangible benefits associated with avoided fear and suffering" that result from the absence of disease. While it is important to rescue children from other forms of distress, disease prevention, detection, and treatment should not be selected at the expense of eradication. It is both prudent and ethically justified to employ all of these strategies to achieve better health for all.

One may further distinguish between "hard rescues" and "easy rescues" (Hawkins 2006) and argue that disease eradication amounts to a hard rescue that imposes excessive burden. Are we not morally obliged to pursue easier rescues? This objection largely depends on two assumptions shown to be false. First, it assumes that burden is disproportionately shouldered by any one agent, when disease eradication is generally a global effort. In fact, burden can be distributed so that it is not excessively taxing for any particular agent, and results on balance to the benefits of completing the rescue outweighing the collective burden. Second, this objection also assumes that objective criteria can define easy rescues. The extent to which a rescue may be considered "easy" or "hard" depends on context and mitigating factors that are dynamic and subject to change with evolving circumstances. Thus, what might be considered a hard rescue may shift and become an easy rescue, and vice versa. In 2003, the boycott of polio vaccination in northern Nigeria owing to sociopolitical reasons resulted in a surge of polio cases that led to exportation of the virus and a global outbreak. For a while, it would seem that it was simply too hard to contain polio under such challenging circumstances, and all hope of eradication was evaporating with the report of each new case (Kaufmann and Feldbaum 2009). However, as a result of a major infusion of resources and a great deal of diplomacy and determination, the boycott came to an end and the polio outbreak was brought under control. Nigeria might have appeared to be a hard rescue at the time, but it has since continued to report record-low levels of poliovirus transmission among the countries where polio remains endemic.[6]

Duty to Future Generations

A duty to spare future generations the harms associated with disease provides additional ethical motivation to pursue eradication. As previously argued, "obligations to future generations are difficult to define and may be limited, but if preventing harm is a moral duty, there may be a chain of obligation that persists through generations and applies to circumstances where present generations could have meaningful impact" (Emerson and Singer 2010). Underpinning Hans Jonas influential ethic of responsibility is the belief that actions have no geospatial boundaries, so that present activities have impact in the future and in the entire world space (Jonas 1984). As such, it is essential to reflect on what responsibilities one has in relation to future people. This line of argument is often employed to inspire efforts to protect the environment against degradation, so that future generations can inherit a healthy planet. In the context of health, globalization may exacerbate inequities (Chen and Berlinguer 2001); thus it is important to think about which public health intervention will promote health for all. In this respect, disease eradication serves this goal by ensuring that future generations are free from disease, even while members of the present generation must bear its burden to some degree.

Counter Considerations

A common criticism against claims of duties to future generations is that such duties cannot be justified at the expense of duties owed to the present generation. However, disease eradication presents a unique opportunity and example of how duties to present and future generations are not in conflict. The successful eradication of disease, in effect, rescues present and future individuals alike.

An objection may also be raised that allowing a supposed duty to future generations to influence public health policy is imprudent since the legitimacy of this duty is disputed. The critique centers on whether it is logically coherent to speak of duties to future, nonexistent individuals for whom we would have to ascribe rights. This objection, however, is not compelling; as noted above, there may be duties to others in the absence of correlative rights. Moreover, there is no logical inconsistency, as Surber (1977) argues, "with including future as well as present individuals under the notion of a person as a moral agent who can make legitimate moral demands upon us."

---

[6] In 2010, Nigeria recorded a total of 21 cases, representing a 95% decrease in cases from 2009 (388 cases).

A persuasive account of why we ought to be moved by duties to future generations is given by philosopher Martin Golding (1972), who introduces the idea of a "moral community" and grounds duties in the idea of a common conception of the good, viz. a good for others which is likewise good for me (Surber 1977). Golding calls this shared conception of the good a "social ideal," and to the extent that it is relevant to future individuals, it implies their membership in our moral community to whom we have obligations. If we apply this understanding to the context of disease eradication, we find that freedom from disease is a social ideal of relevance across generations. And insofar as being in a moral community involves interest in the welfare of others, I am moved by my duties to future individuals because their interests coincide with my own.

Global Public Goods

> Where it is feasible, disease eradication (for diseases
> of global scope) can therefore be seen as a GPG…
> —D. Woodward and R. D. Smith (2003:25)

Conceptualizing health as a global public good is nowadays generally uncontroversial. In the scholarly literature we find many comprehensive analyses on the subject (see Woodward and Smith 2003; Barrett 2007), and several advance disease eradication as an example of a global public good. Public goods are defined as goods that are both nonexcludable and nonrivalrous, viz. consumption by one does not preclude consumption by others, and no one is excluded from consumption of the good. Global public goods feature these characteristics, and additionally transcend national borders (i.e., they are global in scope). Woodward and Smith (2003) further qualify that the cross-national characteristic must involve more than two nations, with at least one outside of the traditional regional grouping. Public goods involving two or three close neighbors are considered localized or regional public goods. While there are many interesting normative dimensions to the idea of global public goods and their provision, here we shall briefly consider the ethical implications of defining eradication as a global public good in this way. Specifically, we want to examine whether the eradication of a disease that does not meet the "global scope" criterion, may in other respects be considered a global public good.

Every year there are approximately 250 million cases of malaria resulting in nearly one million deaths—affecting mostly children. Lymphatic filariasis (LF) is also a mosquito-borne disease, but it is not a "killer'" like malaria. Rather, it is known for causing permanent and long-term disability in its victims, and recognizable by the characteristic swollen limbs. Other features that these two diseases have in common include the following: they cause tremendous human suffering; they have an impact on economic development by disabling their victims; are both deemed potentially eradicable;[7] and may not be global in scope at a given time. This latter feature is relevant, since it disqualifies the eradication of malaria or LF from being considered a global public good, placing it as a regional public good. Why is this disqualification ethically significant? Because global public goods are supposed to be universally desired (Barrett 2007), and we can assume, therefore, that they are globally pursued. However, we cannot assume the same about regional public goods; it follows that these goods are locally desired and pursued. Scott Barrett (2007) asks, "Why should we care if global public goods are provided?" The question is telling; global public goods are underprovided and need incentive for provision. If this is true, what are the odds of providing for regional public goods, which presumably are not universally desired? We surmise that provision of such goods presents a serious challenge, since those outside of the affected regions have little incentive to pursue goods that appear to be of slight relevance to them. In short, this characterization of goods potentially undermines global motivation to pursue the eradication of diseases that affect only those in a few parts of the world.

In the context of eradication, distinguishing goods on the basis of geography may be ethically problematic. If it is only the eradication of disease deemed global in scope that is considered a global public good, there may not be sufficient motivation from the global community to pursue the eradication of regionally confined diseases. This would result in further neglect of diseases that almost exclusively affect the poor in low-to-middle income countries. Limiting global public goods by geography also fails to appreciate that eradication of diseases such as malaria and LF would have global impact, even if they are not global in scope; the economic implications alone would extend far beyond regional borders. Finally, there are morally relevant aspects of eradication such as the promotion of solidarity and social justice that are of significance to the entire global community. The "local" eradication of disease contributes to global health equity.[8] Therefore, it is sensible to extend the notion of disease eradication as a global public good to the eradication of all diseases, whether they are national, regional, or global.

Conclusion

The importance of considering ethical arguments in global public health decision making should not be underestimated. Ethical arguments can balance both moral and nonmoral judgments about a course of action and illuminate the ethical motivation that underlies our reasoning. The duty to rescue, duty

---

[7] Note, however, that consensus is lacking on whether malaria is currently an eradicable disease.

[8] Note that the revised definitions of eradication and elimination in this volume are consistent with an understanding of "regional" eradication (see Cochi and Dowdle, this volume).

to future generations, and the idea of disease eradication as a global public good offer compelling ethical arguments in support of disease eradication. The implication is that these arguments ought to be considered in the balance of reasons that inform decisions about whether or not to pursue eradication.

Acknowledgments

The author is grateful to Jocalyn Clark and an anonymous reviewer for helpful comments on an earlier draft of the manuscript, and to Peter Singer and participants of the Ernst Strüngmann Forum for constructive feedback on the background paper.

9

Economic Evaluation of the Benefits and Costs of Disease Elimination and Eradication Initiatives

Kimberly M. Thompson and Radboud J. Duintjer Tebbens

Abstract

As health care costs continue to increase, economic evaluations of public health interventions play an increasingly important role in resource allocation decisions. In some cases, opportunities exist to eliminate and eradicate some diseases; such efforts typically require committing significant amounts of financial resources, with eradication also requiring international cooperation and coordination. Are investments in disease elimination or eradication worthwhile? How can we evaluate the economics of elimination and eradication efforts? What methodological issues might warrant special consideration? At a time when global health leaders continue to strive for global eradication of wild polioviruses types 1 and 3 (type 2 eradication occurred in 1999) and guinea worm (dracunculiasis), and to debate other eradication efforts related to measles and malaria, economic analyses can provide important context for the discussions. One of the most significant challenges in conducting economic analyses relates to valuing the direct and indirect benefits of elimination nationally and eradication globally. This chapter discusses the requirements for disease elimination or eradication. It presents the methods and challenges and raises key questions associated with evaluating the economic benefits of disease elimination and eradication.

Introduction

Global spending on health exceeds several trillion US dollars annually (WHO 2007c), and costs continue to increase with the growing global population, development, and improvements in health services and technology. A recent edition of the "State of the World's Vaccines and Immunization" (WHO et al. 2009) highlights the enormous health benefits achieved within the last decade from infectious disease prevention due to increased global investment in immunization. As noted in the report, "immunization remains one of the most cost-effective health interventions...[and] by keeping children healthy, immunization helps extend life expectancy and the time spent on productive activity" (WHO et al. 2009:74). Although the well-recognized benefits of vaccines include improving both the quality and length of life, vaccines cost money to produce and distribute; thus the public health community must make investment cases to support public health commitments to and prioritization of expenditures on vaccines. Economic analyses play a critical role with respect to characterizing the benefits and costs of elimination and eradication initiatives.

In some cases, the use of vaccines and/or other interventions (e.g., the isolation of potentially infected patients) can lead to the elimination or eradication of a human disease (for a discussion on definitions, see Cochi and Dowdle, this volume). Following the cessation of transmission of a disease within national or regional borders, people in the area still generally need to continue to use the vaccine or other intervention to maintain high levels of population immunity, to protect themselves from potential importation of the disease from other countries or regions, and to inhibit the reestablishment of transmission. Going beyond national disease control efforts, elimination and eradication initiatives generally require some level of international coordination and cooperation to ensure that the infections cease to circulate in all populations contemporaneously. Control measures (e.g., vaccination) may still be desirable given the possibility of an unintentional (e.g., accidental laboratory release) or intentional (e.g., bioterrorism attack) reintroduction of the infectious agent; thus, economic analyses of elimination and eradication initiatives should explicitly consider the costs and benefits of activities required to maintain the infection-free and/or disease-free state (Miller et al. 2006; Thompson and Duintjer Tebbens 2007). This may prove challenging, because estimating the post-elimination or post-eradication costs and benefits requires making assumptions about future policies and uncertain risks, and modeling the various potential policy options. We expect, however, that such analyses can play a significant role in informing policies, and we recognize that investment cases will need to consider the different values and perspectives that individual nations or regions may bring to international discussions.

Economists typically evaluate health interventions using cost-effectiveness analysis (CEA) and benefit-cost analysis (BCA). In the context of health economics, existing guidelines attempt to standardize the analytical methods used to assess the incremental impacts of potential new health interventions compared to the current intervention using cost-effectiveness methods (e.g., Gold et al. 1996; WHO 2008a). Although traditional CEA tends to provide a static assessment (i.e., to evaluate the economics by taking a snapshot at a fixed point in time), within the last decade analysts have increasingly recognized the importance of taking a dynamic perspective and combining economic models with infection transmission models (Edmunds et al. 1999; Brisson and Edmunds

2003; Thompson and Duintjer Tebbens 2006; WHO 2008a). However, the dynamics of disease elimination and eradication differ from those of disease control (Duintjer Tebbens and Thompson 2009). Notably, theoretical analyses show that achieving eradication may prove difficult if prevalence of the disease drives demand for vaccine (Geoffard and Philipson 1997) (or by extension, the demand for elimination- or eradication-related control efforts). In the context of evaluating the economics of polio eradication, we demonstrated that as disease incidence drops due to significant investments in vaccination, this could lead to a perception that further investments are not worthwhile and to public demands to shift resources to other interventions, which ultimately could yield both higher costs and cases (Thompson and Duintjer Tebbens 2007). Part of the reason for this perception stems from the fact that cases of disease prevented defy observation: we cannot easily count events that do not happen, but we can easily add up financial costs. Models can play a critical role by bringing transparency to both the benefit and cost sides of the discussion. We reviewed the historical successful and failed efforts to eradicate endemic diseases and demonstrated the real trade-offs associated with changing perceptions and priorities in the context of managing multiple eradicable diseases competing for resources (Duintjer Tebbens and Thompson 2009). Other studies explored eradication in the context of game theoretic approaches (e.g., Barrett 2003, 2004; Barrett and Hoel 2007; Thompson and Duintjer Tebbens 2008b). A recent article (Beutels et al. 2008) emphasized that traditional economic methods fail when assessing the economics of emerging diseases, which may be eliminated or eradicated, in large part due to their inability (a) to develop appropriate infection transmission models given uncertainty about characteristics of the emerging pathogen, (b) to characterize the costs and effectiveness of potential interventions, and (c) to do so rapidly enough to inform urgent decisions (i.e., delaying actions until completion of analyses may mean missing critical opportunities for prevention).

Requirements for Disease Elimination or Eradication

Before considering the value and valuation of disease elimination or eradication, it is important to provide context related to the life cycle of diseases and prerequisites for disease elimination or eradication. In the context of their impact on global human health, we characterize diseases as occurring in the following phases:

1. emerging (initial detection/outbreak of a new disease),
2. epidemic (subsequent outbreaks and spread to other areas),
3. endemic and not controllable (continuing circulation of infectious agent in the absence of control strategies),

4.   endemic and controllable (continuing circulation of infectious agent in the presence of control strategies),
5.   eliminated, and
6.   eradicated.

Countries typically go through these phases at different times, which may blur the distinction of these phases globally.

Although our discussion focuses primarily on diseases in the last phases, efforts to eradicate an emerging disease represent important and valuable opportunities to prevent it from becoming endemic. For example, public health officials successfully detected the emergence of severe acute respiratory syndrome (SARS) and quarantined infectious people despite delayed notification of its emergence in the Guangdong province in China. SARS cases occurred in thirty countries around the world, with the disease establishing chains of transmission in six countries (WHO 2003b). As a result of globally coordinated activities, SARS failed to achieve sustained chains of transmission and disappeared. The significant investment in stopping transmission led to a complete disruption of the chains of transmission for SARS. However, this does not meet the definition of eradication of established human diseases (see Cochi and Dowdle, this volume), because SARS never became established and an uncertain nonhuman reservoir may exist which could lead to reemergence at some point. Still, we emphasize the importance of valuing the ability to stop an emerging disease like SARS from becoming established and thus requiring eradication.

In the case of SARS, impacted areas clearly suffered significant economic losses (GAO 2004). Remarkably, however, no studies currently exist that quantify both the costs incurred and benefits generated by the World Health Organization (WHO), U.S. Centers for Disease Control and Prevention (CDC), and other public health and health system authorities whose efforts collectively stopped SARS before it could become established or endemic. An economic analysis of the use of quarantine to stop the outbreak in Toronto reported cost savings (Gupta et al. 2005). We anticipate that analyses for other countries would show similar results, although requirements for international assistance to support efforts in some countries may necessitate transfers of financial, scientific, and health resources. In our initial efforts to assess the costs and benefits retrospectively, we could not find documentation of the costs incurred by the CDC or WHO, which transferred resources in the form of essential supplies for infection control and teams of specialists. Based on the costs incurred in impacted areas and the threat of a pandemic (i.e., rapid spread of an emerging disease throughout a large part of the world), we hypothesize that economic analyses of the efforts implemented to eradicate SARS would most likely suggest that the efforts represented a cost- and life-saving investment. For example, extrapolating the economic impacts experienced by Toronto to major U.S. urban areas provides some indication that prevention of a SARS outbreak in the United States led to significant savings. The CDC's contributions to the efforts largely came from reallocation of existing resources, albeit with the reallocation of resources implying real opportunity costs associated with using the resources for SARS instead of their original purposes. In this regard, we suggest the need to ensure the existence of sufficient global resources to eradicate any future emerging diseases rapidly before they become endemic. We should expect that emerging diseases may occur in the future, and appreciate the importance of preparedness in our ability to control, eliminate, or eradicate new diseases as they emerge. We also emphasize that in the context of responding to an outbreak, faster is generally better (Thompson et al. 2006). Thus, global health authorities should seek to ensure that proper incentives exist to motivate early detection, reporting, coordination, and action related to the management of emerging diseases.

Since most human diseases of concern emerged long ago (Shulman 2004), they fall into the middle disease phases (i.e., epidemic, endemic, or eliminated), which are the focus of this book (see Cochi and Dowdle, this volume). Although many developed countries have successfully stopped the transmission of some diseases, the same diseases remain endemic in other countries. Different types of infectious agents require different types of interventions and, notably, some types of interventions exist only for a subset of infectious agents (i.e., vaccines or medications currently exist for some diseases but not others). The development and widespread use of antibiotic, antitoxin, and antiviral medications to combat infections significantly reduced their adverse health outcomes, but also created conditions that select for resistant organisms, thus creating new problems.

The development of vaccines represents one of the most important tools for preventing many viral and bacterial vaccine-preventable diseases. Although intentional infection of humans to protect them from disease began many centuries ago in the form of variolation, the concept of vaccination derives from the development of the use of a vaccine made from cowpox to protect people from smallpox (Jenner 1801; Fenner et al. 1988). Edward Jenner's 1801 prophecy that "the annihilation of smallpox—the most dreadful scourge of the human race—will be the final result of this practice" (Jenner 1801:8) did not become reality until nearly 180 years later, when global smallpox eradication was certified in 1979 (Fenner et al. 1988).

In 1988, the World Health Assembly committed to the "elimination of the indigenous transmission of wild poliomyelitis viruses" (World Health Assembly 1988), which led to the launch of the Global Polio Eradication Initiative (GPEI). Following the development and introduction of poliovirus vaccines in the mid-1950s and early 1960s, countries increasingly adopted them for disease control efforts. Czechoslovakia and Cuba documented the absence of indigenous wild poliovirus transmission in 1960 and 1962, respectively (Slonim et al. 1995; Más Lago 1999). The burden of polio disease in the United States dropped rapidly in the 1960s and 1970s, and the United States successfully stopped indigenous circulation of all three types of wild polioviruses in 1979 (Thompson and Duintjer Tebbens 2006; Alexander et al. 2004). In 1985, the Pan American Health Organization (PAHO) resolved to stop indigenous transmission of wild poliovirus in the Americas by 1990, which it achieved in 1991 (Tambini et al. 2006). The GPEI achieved the global eradication of type 2 wild polioviruses shortly before 2000 (WHO 2001c), although the overall eradication initiative seeks to eradicate all three types of wild polioviruses (i.e., polio eradication).

Evaluating the feasibility of elimination or eradication requires consideration of many factors. Countries or regions need to possess the tools required to detect the disease based on a defined classification of identifiable disease symptoms and/or laboratory tests and the tools required to stop the transmission of the disease. For diseases that only involve person-to-person spread (i.e., no vector or other environmental reservoir) this may mean isolation of infected (or potentially infected) individuals, as with SARS. Diseases that involve vectors or environmental media may require activities to control or stop transmission from these sources. This occurs now in the case of the parasitic infection dracunculiasis (guinea worm), which requires isolating humans carrying a worm from water sources. For vaccine-preventable diseases, stopping transmission occurs once a population achieves a sufficiently high level of overall immunity (i.e., herd or population immunity) that stops the transmission of infection. The feasibility of stopping transmission depends on the ability of the vaccine to provide at least partial protection from infection, access to sufficient quantities of the vaccine required, an effective vaccine delivery system, absence of nonhuman reservoirs, and maintaining levels of population immunity to transmission of infections sufficient to stop transmission throughout the nation or region. For diseases that we can potentially stop by using nonvaccine interventions, including pharmaceutical products, feasibility depends on sufficient quantities of the intervention and effective use throughout the nation or region. In general, success depends on a functional health system or a dedicated program that can coordinate and manage national and/ or regional resources and continue vigilant disease surveillance as well as any efforts required to avoid importations. Sustained success requires prohibiting any infections that get imported from establishing new chains of transmission by responding quickly and effectively.

The prerequisites for global eradication include the ability to eradicate disease from all countries contemporaneously and a global commitment to coordinate efforts. Eradication initiatives will generally require the establishment and maintenance of a global disease surveillance system, which requires significant investment of resources and may require sharing and transfer of both technologies and other resources.

Valuation of Disease Elimination and Eradication

Economic analyses for infectious diseases must begin by considering the disease phase and feasibility, as discussed in the previous section. We emphasize that traditional economic methods will encounter significant challenges when assessing the economics of emerging diseases (Beutels et al. 2008), but analysts should seek, whenever possible, to evaluate the specific interventions required to eliminate an emerging disease before it becomes endemic. Economic assessments must identify potential interventions, quantify the costs of the interventions, and estimate the health benefits associated with their implementation. In the context of an emerging disease, for which the nature and ability to transmit represent significant uncertainties, analysts face significant challenges in forecasting the potential burdens of disease (with or without any interventions) and in identifying interventions to evaluate. Adding to these difficulties, national economic evaluations should also attempt to consider the positive externalities for other countries associated with eradication in the context of their national activities (i.e., failure to contain and stop transmission will lead to exportation to other countries that will incur costs to fight it, and many of these countries might be willing to pay significant amounts to prevent importation). Thus, in the context of an economic analysis to stop an emerging disease, the economics of eradication represent a relevant consideration; countries will need to create appropriate mechanisms to transfer all required resources from the countries willing to share available required resources to the countries which need them. This may imply incurring transaction costs associated with the transfer of resources, mobilizing financial resources and supplies, political negotiations for access to impacted areas, and managing issues related to ownership of scientific information and data generated by scientific and operational experts brought in to help. Based on the experience with SARS, some of this occurs already because of existing relationships between national and global health authorities that facilitate transactions and reduce some of these costs. However, the process remains somewhat informal, and consideration of transaction costs may represent an important step. By including the example of SARS, efforts taken to stop transmission of a disease before it becomes established represent a very valuable, important, and often-overlooked form of disease eradication activities. Thus, for an emerging disease, national economic analyses of transmission cessation activities need to be framed to include both the national and global perspectives, given large expected values of some countries (e.g., high-income countries) to invest in global prevention of establishment of the emerging disease.

For established diseases, we anticipate that economists will evaluate interventions to achieve national or regional disease elimination using standard CEA and BCA methods, by comparing the incremental costs and benefits of the elimination interventions to the base case comparator. These analyses require evaluation of both the benefits and costs. A typical CEA focuses on estimation of the incremental cost-effectiveness ratio (ICER) in monetary units (e.g., USD) per health outcome of the intervention (i) (i.e., the elimination or eradication initiative) compared to the comparator (c) (i.e., the base case or status quo):

$$ICER(i,c) = \frac{\sum_{j=t_0}^{t}\left[\left(C_{j,i} - C_{j,c} - \left(H_{j,c} - H_{j,i}\right)T\right)/\left(1+\delta\right)^{j-t_0}\right]}{\sum_{j=t_0}^{t}\left[\left(H_{j,c} - H_{j,i}\right)/\left(1+\delta\right)^{j-t_0}\right]} \qquad (9.1)$$

where $C_{j,p}$ represents costs for policy scenario p (with p either i or c) during year j; $H_{j,p}$ is the incidence of health outcome for policy scenario p during year j; T describes the direct treatment costs per unit of health outcome; δ is the discount rate; t_0 represents the starting time of implementation of the intervention; and t signifies the end time of the analytical time horizon (typically chosen such that outcomes beyond time t have little impact on overall outcome due to discounting)

Many interventions impact both mortality and morbidity; thus CEA guidelines focus on reporting the health outcomes in the form of disability- or quality-adjusted life years (i.e., DALYs or QALYs) (WHO 2008a). Estimation of ICERs requires inclusion of the average treatment cost per case (T) to capture the real financial savings associated with not treating the prevented health outcomes. However, interpretation of the ICER and desirability of investing in the intervention require implicit valuation of the health outcomes estimated in the denominator (i.e., the decision maker must judge the cost-effectiveness and acceptability of a certain cost per health outcome determined by the CEA). The use of BCA depends on making the valuation of the denominator explicit (i.e., including an estimate of the monetary value or shadow price associated with the health outcomes saved). Thus, a typical BCA focuses on estimating the incremental net benefits (INB) in dollars associated with implementing the intervention (i) compared to the base case comparator (c):

$$INB(i,c) = \sum_{j=t_0}^{t}\left[\left(\left(H_{j,c} - H_{j,i}\right)\left(T+W\right) - \left(C_{j,i} - C_{j,c}\right)\right)/\left(1+\delta\right)^{j-t_0}\right] \qquad (9.2)$$

where W represents the societal willingness-to-pay per unit of health outcome saved for indirect benefits to society associated with productivity gains, avoided pain and suffering, and other avoided burdens (not including direct treatment costs, T).

Challenges arise with respect to estimating all components of these equations. Estimating costs typically requires extrapolation from limited data for the intervention and the comparator, and estimating benefits typically requires disease modeling and extrapolation. All aspects of the valuation present difficult questions, with selection of the discount rate, time horizon, perspective, and framing recognized as important choices. Despite decades of recognition of the limited data for valuation (e.g., Creese and Henderson 1980; Cutting 1980), these critical inputs for economic analyses remain highly uncertain. Challenges arise with respect to characterizing both the direct and the indirect benefits. Direct benefits include reductions in mortality and morbidity, which we typically estimate using both data and models, and the associated saved treatment costs, which must be monetized. Indirect benefits include "intangibles" like avoided pain, suffering, and fear, productivity gains associated with family members no longer needing to provide care, and other positive externalities (e.g., reduced disruption of the health care system from disease outbreaks no longer occurring). One method for capturing the indirect benefits uses a value for willingness-to-pay per DALY saved on the order of the average annual gross national income as a best estimate, assuming this captures the real human capital costs associated with losses in productivity due to disability (Hutubessy et al. 2003; WHO 2001b, 2008a). This approach recognizes the large differences that exist in values, preferences, and abilities to spend resources in countries of different income levels. Given that valuation inputs remain highly uncertain and difficult to quantify and that this approach only captures the real productivity losses and not the intangible components of the willingness-to-pay, analysts typically consider a wide range of potential values in sensitivity analyses, with upper bounds of up to three times the average annual gross national income per DALY (WHO 2001b).

Challenges also arise with respect to the time horizon and other framing assumptions that determine the scope of the model (e.g., the choice of t_0, t, and δ in Eqs. 9.1, 9.2), which analysts similarly explore in sensitivity analyses. We demonstrated that choices related to framing significantly influence the economic estimates of historical polio control and elimination activities in the United States (Thompson and Duintjer Tebbens 2006). The discount rate (or rate of time preference) represents an area of ongoing discussion and debate in economics (Gravelle and Smith 2001; Parsonage and Neuburger 1992; van Hout 1998). Although existing guidelines suggest the use of a relatively low discount rate (e.g., 3%) for both future monetary and health outcomes (WHO 2008a; Gold et al. 1996), the choice of the discount rate can significantly impact economic results (WHO 2008a). These issues represent important considerations in economic assessments for elimination and eradication initiatives. Since interventions often continue due to importation risks, we expect an even greater impact in the context of evaluating global eradication efforts, which may consider cessation of the interventions given the absence of any globally circulating infections or disease.

Valuation of Global Eradication

Remarkably, relatively little literature exists related to the economic evaluation of global disease eradication successes. Barrett (2006) and Miller et al.

(2006) present highly favorable economics of the 1967 Intensified Smallpox Eradication Programme, based on historical data (Fenner et al. 1988) and the economic benefits received by the entire world compared to the costs paid by the developed countries that provided international funding. Including the costs paid by the endemic countries (i.e., 31 countries, representing the nearly one billion people that were still reporting cases of smallpox in 1967) decreases the estimated benefit/cost ratio by approximately a factor of 3 (Miller et al. 2006). Even with these costs, the Intensified Smallpox Eradication Programme remains a good global investment based on the benefit/cost ratio, with the endemic countries experiencing a significantly larger proportion of the benefits. We could not find any published economic analyses related to smallpox eradication that follow current guidelines for economic analysis or consider other parts of (or the entire) time horizon between Jenner's vision of smallpox eradication and the actual achievement nearly 180 years later. We also could not find any analyses that quantified the global economics of cessation of transmission of an emerging disease, like for SARS. We found no economic analysis of the global eradication of wild poliovirus type 2, which occurred as part of the GPEI's effort to eradicate all three types of wild polioviruses.

We recently completed an economic analysis of the costs and benefits of the GPEI (Duintjer Tebbens et al. 2011) based on the current status of the program and consideration of post-eradication risk management policies (Thompson et al. 2008; Duintjer Tebbens et al. 2008). Although polio eradication, defined as the complete global disruption of transmission of all three types of wild polioviruses, remains an ongoing effort, the analysis suggests significant benefits associated with the GPEI. Several challenges and insights emerge from that analysis.

First, evaluating the economics of global eradication depends on estimating the number of endemic countries at the time the global eradication initiative starts and appropriately attributing the costs and benefits based on the state of the world at the outset of the initiative. For example, both global smallpox eradication and global polio eradication began following substantial reductions in the incidence of smallpox and polio diseases globally, although the amount of reduction varied considerably: 31 countries with less than 1 billion people living in these countries endemic for the one serotype of smallpox at the launch of the Intensified Smallpox Eradication Programme compared to more than 125 countries with more than 4.5 billion people living in these countries endemic for the three serotypes of wild polioviruses at the launch of the GPEI. With respect to current discussions of measles eradication, we note that significant progress toward elimination and eradication by many nations and WHO regions based on current goals may mean that a relatively small fraction of countries will ultimately directly benefit from a global eradication initiative, although ensuring effective coordination to achieve eradication may require its creation. Nevertheless, the indirect benefits may extend to all countries if global eradication leads to a significant reduction in importation outbreaks or enables eventual cessation of vaccination. The different relative starting points mean that we cannot compare the economics of different eradication efforts directly, although estimates of the net benefits from BCAs for any eradication effort should suffice to indicate the value of the initiative. Based on our modeling, performing CEAs for global eradication initiatives does not make sense given the large differences in the valuation and costs that exist for countries of different income levels. This occurs because analysts often can only provide appropriate estimates of ICERs for individual countries or countries grouped in a similar income level. Providing an "average" ICER for a global eradication effort aggregated at the global level will yield a result that national leaders will find difficult to evaluate, because they will most likely want to compare it to the ICERs for interventions that they undertake nationally. In our analyses of global policies, for which some readers might expect to see global ICERs (Thompson et al. 2008; Duintjer Tebbens et al. 2011), we reported ICERs stratified by income level to provide some indication of the large variability in estimates; we intentionally did not report a global ICER since it could mislead some decision makers by making them see either a significantly smaller or larger ICER than would in fact represent their country. We emphasize that income-level averaged ICERs may suffice to provide an indication of the variability for global analyses, but analysts would need to report national ICERs to support discussion of national and possibly also regional policy discussions. Given the highly variable values and preferences that occur over income levels, national leaders should compare an ICER in $/DALY to their national GNI or GDP per capita (WHO 2008a). However, this means that they need ICERs that reflect the appropriate costs for their country. BCA does not run into these issues because the valuation should occur explicitly as part of the process. Consequently, we believe that economic analyses of eradication initiatives should focus on providing BCA results. Any global eradication analysis will need to address the framing issue of determining the level of stratification required to communicate effectively to decision makers and key stakeholders.

Second, economic analyses must consider the dynamic nature of the eradication process, because countries may disrupt transmission at different times and those that stopped transmission must maintain disruption until all countries contemporaneously disrupt transmission. Models considering the dynamics of disease eradication suggest that the economically optimal path toward eradication involves strong coordination and rapid achievement of this goal (Barrett and Hoel 2007; Duintjer Tebbens and Thompson 2009). However, the economics of stopping transmission may only appear attractive in some countries initially (e.g., those with high health care expenditures and conditions that do not favor transmission of the infectious agent). For example, the costs of the intervention may decrease with time due to economies of scale associated with increased adoption and optimization of production processes. In addition, global eradication may become economically preferable to merely controlling the disease in countries experiencing continued transmission after a critical number of countries control or stop their transmission. This occurs because the risks of importation and the expected time until global eradication decrease, which implies fewer years of intensive efforts required to achieve and maintain national activities (Barrett and Hoel 2007). Failing to consider the dynamics of the process and the costs of delays may lead to an underestimation of the costs of global eradication. This can easily occur because estimating the costs of global eradication depends on making assumptions about national and global activities. We note that developing the types of integrated models needed to support policy considerations (e.g., Thompson et al. 2008; Duintjer Tebbens et al. 2008) may require consideration of many factors and careful documentation of the options (e.g., Sangrujee et al. 2003), risks (e.g., Duintjer Tebbens et al. 2006a), costs (e.g., Duintjer Tebbens et al. 2006b), and dynamics (e.g., Duintjer Tebbens et al. 2005). Experience shows that such forecast activities may not always go as planned. For example, in spite of the global commitment to eradicate wild polioviruses in 1988, some large countries and regions did not begin the necessary vaccination and surveillance efforts until very shortly before the year 2000 (Aylward et al. 2003). Characterizing the costs as a function of time also requires addressing the reality that all countries will need to pay costs associated with achieving global eradication until it occurs, which generally implies relatively large costs for the "last mile" or final stages. We emphasize that an important mismatch may occur during the final stages of global eradication, because costs tend to be relatively high while the number of visible cases is relatively low. During this time communication efforts will need to emphasize that the investment of the high costs means the prevention of a large number of cases.

Third, the costs of post-eradication activities may represent a significant consideration. For example, in the context of polio eradication, some countries may choose to continue to use or switch to using the more expensive inactivated poliovirus vaccine for routine vaccination to lower their risks of outbreaks from potential failures of containment or due to circulating live oral poliovirus vaccine viruses (Thompson et al. 2008). Although the cessation of vaccination and/or other disease control efforts may represent major economic dividends of an eradication initiative, we emphasize that economists must carefully assess post-eradication activities and consider different scenarios in the face of different potential future policies (Thompson et al. 2008; Barrett 2010).

Fourth, for any incremental economic analysis for disease eradication, analysts must compare at least one hypothetical scenario. For example, in the context of evaluating the benefits of polio eradication, we compared the actual GPEI to a scenario representing the alternative world with only routine vaccination (Duintjer Tebbens et al. 2011). Selection of the appropriate comparator for analysis can significantly influence the results and the insights associated with the analysis. One of the most challenging aspects of comparator forecasts relates to assumptions about the intervention over time. For example, what assumptions make sense for routine immunization rates: will they go up, go down, or stay constant over time?

Fifth, many of the choices related to the time horizon, time preferences, and framing can significantly impact the analysis and results (e.g., the choice of t_0, t, and δ in Eqs. 9.1, 9.2, with the modification that t_0 = starting time of implementation of the global eradication effort). Consideration of the discount rate for eradication initiatives raises interesting issues. Without discounting, the prevention of future cases extends to all future generations, which could theoretically imply infinite benefits and the need for an infinite time horizon (or a time horizon that theoretically goes until the uncertain time when the last human being on Earth dies). With discounting, the benefits to future generations disappear at some point in the analysis. The main issue this raises relates to intergenerational considerations, because some of the people who benefit from elimination or eradication initiatives undertaken now will not incur costs of the initiatives, although they benefit and they might be willing to pay such costs. Future generations might strongly prefer for current generations to address eradication instead of extending the burden of disease into the future, but they cannot express their preferences. We expect that economists will continue to perform baseline analyses using relatively low discount rates and present the results for a range of discount rates in sensitivity analyses, but that discussion about this issue will continue.

Finally, methods to estimate the indirect benefits continue to require development and need greater application with respect to disease elimination and eradication initiatives. Quantifying the benefits of a healthier population with respect to productivity and human capital represent significant challenges, and a large part of the value that societies place on health may depend on whether people perceive preventable cases of disease and disability as the norm (i.e., acceptable by default) or not. Disease elimination and eradication initiatives can fundamentally change expectations about health, because once people recognize the possibility of controlling or stopping a disease, this can lead to demands for public disease prevention initiatives. The value of preventing disease and disability in individuals impacts society, because societal resources used for treatment become available for other uses. For example, with effective measles vaccination efforts, the space required for measles wards in hospitals becomes available for treating patients with other diseases. Widespread vaccination for polio quickly led to the end of large rooms filled with iron lungs in hospitals. Thus, polio vaccination meant not only savings of treatment costs for the individual patients, but also big savings for the overall health system. Healthier children also mean more productive families, because caring for disabled family members takes people out of the workforce and uses family resources. Although economists attempt to capture indirect benefits using willingness-to-pay estimates, more current and future research will need to develop these methods further and ensure that they capture all of the benefits, including those that span generations.

Discussion

Although economic analyses provide important information for disease elimination and eradication decisions, analysts encounter challenges preparing them and decision makers face challenges using their results. Economic analyses also represent only one consideration. The option to stop a disease from causing adverse health outcomes permanently into the future implies the opportunity to prevent any future human suffering caused by the disease, and this raises ethical and other considerations (Emerson, this volume; Emerson and Singer 2010).

With respect to the use of economic analysis results, we note that many discussions focus on opportunity costs, because some real resources used for one effort cannot be used for another. The need to pay relatively high costs for a short period of time to achieve eradication and receive long-term benefits often leads to discussions about the opportunity costs associated with the use of the resources during the "last mile" and to suggestions for potential better short-term purposes. We emphasize that opportunity costs require careful consideration for all potential uses. Clearly if a better opportunity exists, based on a rigorous analysis, and no means exist for mobilizing additional resources, then societies must make difficult choices. However, arguments about better opportunities need to show that the alternative use of the resources truly leads to an improvement (i.e., lower costs and lower DALYs lost overall in the short and long term). Thus, consideration of opportunity costs should include not only the potential alternative uses of the resources in the short term, but also the implications of failing to eradicate a disease, and thus incurring ongoing costs for disease control into the long term, because countries will continue to incur such costs. Ignoring these opportunity costs does not make them go away.

The dynamics of optimizing the management of multiple diseases represents an important area for modeling (Duintjer Tebbens and Thompson 2009), particularly because intuition about opportunities may become biased by focusing on cases occurring instead of on the cost-effectiveness of options. Arguments that eradication initiatives represent unreasonable expenses in an absolute sense (e.g., we cannot afford to spend billions of dollars to eradicate a disease) need to consider the context of how such global health projects fit into the context of other major societal projects (Thompson and Duintjer Tebbens 2008b), for which their absolute costs and performance seem favorable. More importantly, we suggest that from an economic perspective, the focus should remain on whether the effort provides net benefits. For a vaccine-preventable disease, the notion that we can invest significantly in building up population immunity as part of an eradication effort and then stop investing prior to achieving eradication without losing any ground represents a logical fallacy. Such an argument fails to appreciate that the true value of an eradication effort derives from the population immunity provided by the vaccine, which protects people from the disease. This protection represents a real value. In all cases, efforts to validate analyses and evaluate progress should provide feedback as to whether resource uses represented cost-effective investments that yield net benefits. We also note that those who suggest better opportunities for elimination or eradication funds should recognize that some of the resources might not exist were it not for the goal of disease eradication (i.e., some sources of funding might provide resources to support some types of goals, but not others, and not all funding is fungible).

One of our main insights from reviewing the economics of disease elimination and eradication initiatives relates to the issue that, in the context of global health, eradication initiatives may represent an activity for which an increase in societal investments could lead to significantly more benefits. One interpretation of the concept that we could potentially eradicate multiple diseases, but that we lack resources to do so, is that global health leaders may not appreciate the significant economic benefits of eradication. Notably, the issue of insufficient financial resources threatened smallpox eradication and continues to threaten polio eradication. Unlike other major projects to develop public goods that typically involve public financing, disease eradication initiatives currently depend on raising all of the funds required up front. Part of the challenge for disease eradication may derive from the difficulty that arises in health systems and the public recognizing the savings associated with not incurring disease and not paying the associated treatment costs. Economic and disease modeling can play an important role in helping to make these more clear, and this may be particularly critical when public perceptions focus on the small number of eradication intervention-related adverse events in the absence of large amounts of disease incidence. Another interpretation of the lack of resources to eradicate diseases is that economic analyses need to provide more assessments with respect to making the investment case for disease control, elimination, and eradication efforts. We suggest that investment cases can and should play a much greater role.

Conclusion

Economic analyses can offer important insights related to disease elimination and eradication initiatives. However, analysts must address a number of challenges before the estimates they provide will truly assist decision makers. The valuation of direct and indirect benefits represents an important area for additional research, particularly related to framing the analysis. Selection of the time horizon, the starting point with respect to the scale of the elimination or eradication initiative, and time preference values may significantly impact the results of the analysis. Sensitivity analyses should provide a strategy for analysts to explore the impacts of different possible choices. Additional research may help analysts better quantify time and intergenerational preferences for all economic analyses of elimination and eradication initiatives. For specific eradication investment cases, we expect that analysts will need to invest in obtaining the best available estimates of the willingness-to-pay for indirect benefits as they move more toward a BCA approach. Finally, global eradication initiatives will need to address the reality of large differences in the economics for different countries.

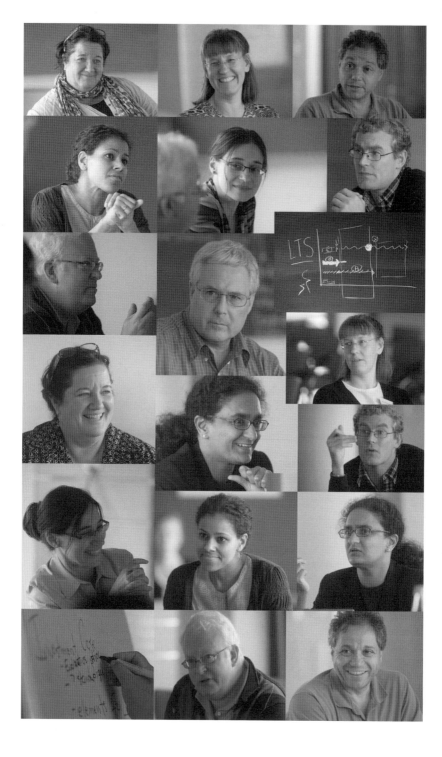

10

Group Report: Developing an Eradication Investment Case

Kimberly M. Thompson, Regina Rabinovich,
Lesong Conteh, Claudia I. Emerson, B. Fenton Hall,
Peter A. Singer, Maya Vijayaraghavan, and Damian G. Walker

Abstract

Eradication initiatives offer important opportunities to provide global as well as intergenerational health benefits. Humankind should aspire to the eradication of diseases; however, the decision to commit to an eradication goal should derive from careful consideration of the evidence base and a thorough discussion of the benefits, risks, and costs of eradication compared to the status quo. This chapter discusses the need to develop an eradication investment case (EIC) as a tool to support the decision-making process involved in launching an eradication initiative.

Eradication initiatives, like other major societal investments (e.g., capital and infrastructure investments), require careful and deliberate conception and management. Benefits from eradication may include the public good of intergenerational health and associated productivity gains and/or economic savings. However, like other major projects, eradication initiatives represent resource-intensive efforts with associated opportunity costs.

Proponents of future eradication initiatives should develop an investment case prior to launch. Critical elements of an EIC are discussed, and the need to standardize the methodology to the greatest extent possible is identified. Since no single overarching decision-making body currently exists to demand and review EICs, an analytic-deliberative process must be developed.

The EIC should support and inform deliberations and decisions made by national health leaders at the World Health Assembly and elsewhere, as they consider a global commitment to an eradication goal. An EIC will also stimulate the development of a financial plan, which will provide details about financing the initiative, as stakeholders evaluate the choice to commit to an eradication goal. The EIC will not, however, include the financial or fundraising plan. Innovation should lead to the creation of additional mechanisms to finance eradication initiatives, perhaps including the use of an "eradication bond." Issues of phasing and timing of multiple eradication initiatives are discussed, as is the need to consider potential synergies of eradication initiatives and opportunities to diversify the disease eradication portfolio.

Introduction

The eradication of a disease offers important opportunities for society, and humankind should aspire to this goal. The eradication of smallpox and the interruption of SARS virus transmission that emerged in 2002, represent significant accomplishments, from which humankind continues to benefit. Eradication initiatives require significant commitments, including major investments of economic and sociopolitical capital. Thus, the decision to commit to an eradication goal should derive from careful consideration of the evidence base and a thorough discussion of the benefits, risks, and costs of eradication compared to the status quo.[1] This chapter discusses the need to develop an eradication investment case (EIC) as a tool to support the decision-making process involved in launching an eradication initiative.

Although decisions to launch past and ongoing eradication initiatives occurred without the benefit of an EIC, we learned from these experiences about the importance of managing expectations better throughout the process. We believe that the EIC will enable this to occur by establishing clear expectations at the outset.

The EIC will serve as a tool that facilitates rigorous evaluation by stakeholders during the decision-making process as they evaluate the choice to move from the base case comparator (i.e., some form of control) to eradication of a specific disease, with full consideration of what this global commitment entails. The EIC provides the context and information needed to support the deliberations of international health leaders and other key stakeholders; it synthesizes all of the information relevant to the choice, taking as a starting point that eradication represents a biologically and technically feasible option (see Strebel et al., this volume). We propose that the EIC include discussion of the global burden of disease; expected benefits, risks, and costs of the eradication and comparator options; social, political, and economic challenges; ethical considerations; and operational and other research needs. An EIC will apply to a specific disease, and for that disease it will address the question: What are the current options related to eradication and control, based on complete characterization and quantification of the risks, costs, benefits, and discussion of qualitative considerations of eradication and control options at the global level? Ideally, when eradication emerges as the best option for multiple diseases, the collection of EICs developed for each disease would inform decisions about phasing coordinated eradication activities to optimize efforts in the context of resource constraints (e.g., financial, political will, capacity), and encourage discussion of the impact on the overall eradicable disease portfolio. We anticipate the ongoing management of multiple eradicable diseases

---

[1] Status quo represents baseline expectations of the current situation and path, whereas when projecting future trajectories, analysts need to consider more than one possibility (e.g., the current situation could remain unchanged, improve, or worsen).

at the same time, and we refer to the set of all potentially eradicable diseases as the eradicable disease portfolio. Managing the eradicable disease portfolio could lead to discussions about the need to challenge any constraints that drive suboptimal management. However, before we can combine and explore EICs for multiple diseases, we need to create an expectation for their development, standardization (to the extent possible), and use.

Stakeholders

Numerous stakeholders would benefit from an EIC. For example, when evaluating the possible adoption of an eradication goal, national health ministers responsible for considering potential commitments for their individual countries could use the evidence-based EIC to inform their decisions. Once eradication represents the preferred international choice (i.e., when it appears that sufficient global motivation exists for national health leaders and other key stakeholders to make the commitment and cooperate to achieve an eradication goal), the EIC would provide the necessary context to support global health diplomacy. It would facilitate consensus about strategies and targets to achieve eradication by informing other stakeholders involved: global health leaders, potential funding partners and national finance ministers, intervention producers (e.g., pharmaceutical and biotechnology companies that produce vaccines, therapeutic agents, and delivery devices), partners in health systems at multiple levels, community leaders, individual consumers, and opinion leaders from low- and middle-income countries and representatives of affected populations.

The development of an EIC should occur as part of an analytic-deliberative process that involves active consultation with all stakeholders. We suggest that the process itself will ultimately prove as valuable as the final EIC document, because it will characterize demand for eradication in the context of the complex geopolitical environment and result in a concrete plan, which can then form the basis for developing a financial plan.

The responsibility for synthesizing the solid evidence base and developing the EIC will most likely fall on the stakeholders who step forward to propose detailed plans for an eradication effort (i.e., the proponents). The EIC should rely on a standardized methodology (to the extent possible) and undergo extensive review and iteration, as part of the analytic-deliberative process. Developers of the EIC should strive for objectivity and critical evaluation of the evidence base.

Examples of Investment Cases from Other Contexts

Business plans represent a well-established, generic example of an investment case. Typically, a business plan includes a formal statement of goals, a plan of action, an estimate of the costs of the plan, information about the result of the action, and a discussion of challenges. In general, business plans help organizations look ahead and create expectations for future performance, allocate resources, focus on key issues, and identify and prepare for threats and opportunities. The term "business plan" may suggest a for-profit enterprise. Thus, we chose instead the term "investment case," building on Webster's definition, "to make use of for future benefits or advantages," as this reflects the goals inherent in an eradication initiative. This term is widely recognized by global immunization partners as a result of its regular use by the Global Alliance for Vaccines and Immunization (GAVI).

With respect to specific examples of investment cases that might be of relevance to eradication efforts, we discussed the investment cases that the GAVI Alliance currently uses to support decisions related to expanding its eligible vaccine portfolio (GAVI Alliance 2006). Specifically, GAVI requires the development of an investment case that follows guidelines to support its decision about whether or not to include a specific vaccine in its list of vaccines eligible for GAVI funding. At the highest level, the GAVI investment cases focus on disease burden and potential impact, cost-effectiveness, and demand forecasting and supply strategies. The cases recognize that:

1. Accurately characterizing disease burden requires the establishment and maintenance of surveillance systems,
2. Rigorous and accurate demand forecasts are required to send appropriate signals to multinational and emerging vaccine suppliers, and
3. Stakeholders need high-quality estimates of the value of vaccination to address the national, regional, and global burden of disease.

Each GAVI investment case specifically addresses whether the proposed activity aligns with an existing GAVI goal and/or enables achievement of part of its long-term strategy. For example, in the context of recently evaluating and adding rotavirus vaccine to its portfolio, the investment case suggested that adding rotavirus aligned with GAVI's goal to "accelerate the uptake and use of underused and new vaccines and associated technologies and improve vaccine supply security" (GAVI Alliance 2006).

We identified opportunities to adopt some of the GAVI investment case concepts directly into our discussion, but highlighted the need to develop a specific EIC for eradication initiatives to address the unique attributes of the decisions to pursue eradication and to encompass interventions other than vaccines.

Demand for an Eradication Investment Case

In contrast to the GAVI investment case, no single overarching decision-making body currently exists to demand the creation of EICs or to ensure quality and consistency in the evidence that they would provide. The World Health

Assembly (WHA) might serve as the primary source of demand for an EIC in the context of its consideration of a future WHA resolution for an eradication goal. Notably, the WHA offers the most likely forum for discussion by national health leaders about the desirability to cooperate to achieve an eradication goal, and a WHA commitment most likely represents a necessary requirement for the implementation of coordinated eradication initiatives. Thus, the WHA could demand an EIC as it engages in a process to consider an eradication goal, which requires international cooperation, in contrast to an existing control strategy. We do not believe, however, that only the WHA could demand the development of an EIC. Other stakeholders may request initial development of an EIC for a specific disease.

We suggest the potential need to create a new decision-making process tasked with managing the eradication disease portfolio, in partnership with national health leaders, the World Health Organization, and other stakeholders. Although we discussed the desirability of maintaining independence from advocates, we recognize that eradication efforts need leaders, champions, and underwriters, and that without active advocates, progress toward eradication may not occur optimally (i.e., with timing and resource investments made and managed in a way that maximizes the public good). This implies likely involvement of some advocates in the creation of an EIC and the need for a review process as noted above. Potential reviewers could include the International Task Force for Disease Eradication, a consultation panel convened by the WHO or the InterAcademy Medical Panel, open and/or invited commentary, and peer review.

We discussed the challenges of engaging stakeholders at all levels, and identified community engagement as critical to both characterizing demand and ultimately achieving eradication. We also discussed many issues about how and when to best engage communities, which remain unresolved. The EIC should serve as a tool to provide the context for essential communications about why eradication may or may not represent a goal worth pursuing. We expect that cooperation will likely require negotiation with stakeholders at multiple levels. The EIC should serve to help highlight the reasons why countries set out with different perspectives about the value of eradication as it relates to their national concerns, and provide a perspective about whether or not eradication might lead to a better future. While the EIC will present evidence on the global argument for eradicating a disease, we note that it will not focus on evaluating national cases, so countries will need to develop these separately if necessary to support their decision making process.

Recognizing the importance of providing context to ensure that stakeholders use the available evidence as they assess their demand for eradication, we discussed the comparator for any EIC, and noted that the base case (i.e., presumably some form or forms of control) would represent the relevant starting point for an EIC. This could mean starting in relatively different places for different diseases, since nations and regions may vary with respect to the progress made prior to consideration of the EIC for any individual disease and their use of the intervention. Consider, for example, the starting point for smallpox eradication in 1958 with under 1 billion people living in endemic countries versus polio eradication in 1988 with approximately 4.5 billion people living in endemic countries (Thompson and Duintjer Tebbens 2007). In this regard, the EIC should include a discussion about the disease context at the time of the analysis (i.e., description of the status quo and the path leading to it, the current costs of control, and the current burden of disease). The base case should represent the baseline expectations about the current situation and path, but in projecting the future or reconstructing a counterfactual scenario, analysts may need to consider more than one possibility: the current situation could remain unchanged, improve, or worsen, and the past could have been different. A study of the economics of the Global Polio Eradication Initiative (Duintjer Tebbens et al. 2011) provides an example of an analysis that dealt with uncertainty about the past and future when considering the base case comparator and eradication with different potential future post-eradication policies. While we do not expect the EIC to necessarily assess every possible scenario, the analysis should consider the wide range of possibilities; then, if an eradication initiative is launched, those managing the effort should periodically revisit the assumptions in the EIC to update and manage expectations (see Stoever et al., this volume). Analysts may need to consider explicitly the reality that the status quo may not represent the economically optimal level, which could occur in either direction (i.e., currently over- or under-investing from a purely economic perspective). We emphasize that the dynamics, situation, and system require careful consideration, because economic analyses often depend on unrealistic assumptions of equilibrium and/or ignore time, and such analyses will not capture the real time delays that exist in the system. For example, some period of high control will most likely represent a prerequisite to actually achieving an elimination or eradication goal, and a period of low control may reflect real system constraints that exist in producing, procuring, and/or implementing interventions.

Critical Elements of the Eradication Investment Case

Using the GAVI investment case as a model, we derived an initial list of critical elements specific to disease eradication and development of an EIC. We emphasize that several critical elements of the EIC differ from the GAVI model, because the EIC focuses on an analysis related to the cooperation necessary to achieve eradication, and this may involve a large spectrum of vaccine and/or nonvaccine interventions.

The Proposed Investment

- Description of the disease and its global health significance.
- Transparent characterization of the status quo (i.e., the base case), based on historical context and projections for the future path (may involve consideration of multiple possibilities allowing analysts to identify other options and distinguish comparators from potential interventions).
- Articulation of a specific plan for achieving eradication; includes a proposed timeline, projections about how the world will look after eradication is achieved, and discussion of expected post-eradication activities.
- Assessment of the current burden of disease, in terms of relevant morbidity and mortality metrics, using disability-adjusted life years (DALYs) to capture both in the context of a single health metric; discussion of historical trends related to the burden of disease.
- Articulation of the role of ongoing research in achieving eradication.
- Discussion of the current methods and challenges for disease and infection control, including vaccination with various delivery strategies, if applicable, and other interventions used in practice.
- Discussion of the public good obtained by eradication and how this differs from the status quo.
- Discussion of the need for cooperation at the global level to obtain the public good.

Rationale for Investing

- Documentation of sufficient evidence of biological and technical feasibility and review of any relevant evidence related to proof of concept.
- Presentation of evidence of demand for eradication and willingness to cooperate at the global level.
- Projection of burden of disease expected over the time horizon for analysis for the status quo and the eradication effort (based on the specific plan).
- Discussion of anticipated challenges and constraints (ethical, geopolitical, social, economic, epidemiologic, technical and institutional) for the status quo and eradication plan, and strategies to address these.
- Assessment of why existing health systems, stratified by relevant categories or types, have/have not achieved elimination, and discussion of how the global plan integrates and strengthens health systems, with particular emphasis on how planned activities will be achieved in countries with the weakest, most fragile health systems.
- Discussion of anticipated global and national resource requirements for the status quo and eradication plan over the same time horizon for different scenarios.

- Discussion of critical risks associated with attempting to move from control to eradication, including the ethical and social risks.
- Assessment of total costs (including programmatic resources) associated with the status quo and eradication plan (aggregated to the global level and also appropriately disaggregated as needed to address heterogeneity issues), with consideration of the impact of time delays and contingency plans included that explore the potential for cost overruns if the eradication plan does not perform as expected.
- Assessment of health outcomes associated with the status quo and eradication plan (aggregated to the global level and also appropriately disaggregated as needed to address heterogeneity issues).
- Transparent discussion of broader social impacts, including intergenerational benefits, equity (e.g., reaching marginalized populations), and the social value of eradication of disease; that is, lives rescued and worry avoided (e.g., nonexistence value), community morale (the sense "warm glow" of accomplishment).
- Assessments of cost-effectiveness and benefit-cost estimates, including efforts to demonstrate the impacts of explicit choices regarding valuation of health outcomes and nonmonetary benefits and appropriate sensitivity analyses.
- Discussion of projected impacts on demand and supply of the interventions and the effect on prices and availability, considering bottlenecks in the development, distribution, procurement, and/or manufacturing of key materials, at all appropriate and required levels (i.e., global, national, community).
- Discussion of capacity of qualified staff and technical resources.
- Discussion of assumptions about post-eradication plans, including discussion of expected needs for continued intervention, surveillance, commodity stockpiles, and/or outbreak response.

Management and Governance

- Discussion of proposed eradication initiative partnerships and plan for governance.
- Establishment of critical milestones, including any critical decision and action points, and the plan for monitoring, oversight, and evaluation of milestones.
- Assessment of diagnostic tools for monitoring.
- Discussion of the risk management plan for critical ethical, geopolitical, social and other risks.
- Discussion of the operational research plan and the proposed strategy for how operational research would be supported.
- Discussion of the proposed process for active evaluation of any impacts on health systems.

Critical Issues and Standardization of Methods

To promote objectivity and comparability of results, people preparing an EIC should use standardized methods and reporting of information to the extent possible. Key issues for standardization include choices related to managing time preferences in the framing of the analysis and key inputs, such as the discount rate. We raised the issue of using consistent time horizons for post-eradication activities while noting the difficulties associated with forecasting decades into the future. We also discussed the need to characterize different options for the pre- and post-eradication timelines and the importance of developing some standards related to the conduct and presentation of the economic analysis performed to quantify the benefits and costs of eradication and the base case scenarios.

Considerations of ethical issues during the development of an EIC will clarify the potential ethical challenges (Emerson, this volume). Thus we included the requirement of a narrative of the moral value of launching an eradication program with respect to the lives rescued, benefits accrued to future generations, and contribution to the broader public good. The narrative should capture the value of intangible benefits and ensure consideration of benefits that are difficult to quantify. In addition, an EIC must make explicit the anticipated ethical and social risks, and outline a plan to address these, because unattended ethical and social barriers can derail the critical path to success of an eradication program. For example, the 2003 polio vaccination boycott in northern Nigeria occurred, at least in part, as a result of ethical, social, and cultural issues (Kaufmann and Feldbaum 2009); inadequate attention to trust, communication, community ownership, and community engagement emerged as major contributing factors (Obadare 2005). Such experiences teach us that we must seek to anticipate some of the challenges and create early interventions. Thus, as an ethical requirement and an ingredient for success, the EIC should present potential strategies to engage relevant communities and key opinion leaders, as a means of identifying the critical barriers early on and as part of the effort to gain and sustain public support. Public support and willingness to endorse future eradication initiatives may depend on the success of current initiatives. The success of polio eradication may be important with respect to the pursuit of future eradication initiatives and global health efforts more broadly.

In terms of projections, the EIC should clearly articulate critical barriers and the end game. In addition, the EIC should anticipate that the costs of eradication may increase during the final stages, due to the need to access harder-to-reach populations as well as the impact of sustaining high levels of activity globally while coping with delays in achieving milestones. The EIC should create realistic expectations, provide contingency plans, and explore "what-if" scenarios. Once launched, an eradication effort will require ongoing operational research, which the EIC should characterize explicitly.

For issues related to health systems, we determined that eradication programs should not be expected to fix health systems, but that they should create strategies that seek to provide overall net benefits to the extent possible. Thus, an EIC should clearly delineate linkages to the health systems and should seek opportunities to create positive externalities.

In our discussions, a critical issue arose as to whether an eradication plan should prioritize easiest and lowest cost activities first, or address more challenging targets first to demonstrate the possibility of eradication in these places. Tackling relatively easier areas first would help to build momentum, test approaches, and eliminate the disease in geopolitical settings likely to maintain elimination. Waiting to start in the difficult areas, however, will inevitably lead to delays. We suggest that the EIC should explore the impacts of timing decisions and trade-offs by modeling the impacts of various scenarios, which would be used in the context of discussions to develop the implementation and financing plan.

We identified the need for a separate effort to focus specifically on developing a guidance document—one that would develop standards for preparing an EIC. This document would build on the standardized guidelines for economic analyses of vaccine interventions (WHO 2008a) and add to that framework to account specifically for eradication-related issues. With respect to the specific terms of reference for this effort, we discussed the need to standardize EIC methods and presentation of results with respect to the following:

1. The assumptions about time related to the characterization of the ethics and economics of benefit to future generations, prior to and after eradication, and the development of recommendations for the analytical time horizon and discount rate for use in the base case and sensitivity analyses.
2. The precise format for the ethical framework for the analysis and development of a standard set of questions that must be answered in the narrative and any recommended set of key ethical criteria for consideration. This framework could be based on broader considerations, such as the ethical significance of rescue, obligations to future generations, and creation of public goods (Emerson and Singer 2010).
3. The process and dynamics of decision making, and assumptions about how to address barriers.
4. The review process and development of a specific checklist for review.

Process

The EIC will serve as a tool to *facilitate* discussions, but it does not and cannot *make* the decision to commit to an eradication initiative. Development of an EIC will require iteration as part of an analytic-deliberative process.

Stakeholders should actively engage in reviewing drafts and challenging assumptions, prior to finalization of the EIC and its use by global partners and WHA leaders (e.g., in support of a global resolution) or other stakeholders (e.g., to develop a financial plan). We identified potential strategies (e.g., focus groups, surveys) to solicit public opinion and to encourage stakeholder engagement early and often in the process. Stakeholder involvement needs to include a wide range of individuals and voices, preferably at multiple levels; however, early engagement of key national opinion leaders may facilitate more rapid implementation. Implementing a systematic process to engage stakeholders should improve the process, but exactly how to accomplish this remains an area for further research.

Standardized guidelines will ensure that EICs present evidence-based information, and we discussed the need for a rigorous review process involving a broad array of voices and technical experts (e.g., health, economic, programmatic, ethics, policy, implementation). We did not address the issues related to how diseases get selected for development of an EIC in detail, although we expect that the initial list would consider diseases already identified as eradicable (ITFDE 2008).

Financing

The EIC document would make the economic case for eradication or continuance of the status quo. It should identify the expected financial needs, should decision makers choose to pursue eradication, but it would not include the actual financial plan. The EIC would support efforts to prepare a financial plan and seek financing.

The financial needs analysis should anticipate and estimate the expected resources required for national efforts and address the need to identify potential nongovernmental sources of financial support. In this regard, we explored existing and potential strategies for apportioning contributions and discussed the challenges of dealing with free riders that occurs with many public goods. For example, if the financial resources of an initiative depend on grants, then the eradication initiative will need to engage grant-making early in the process. This, in turn, requires a clear delineation of the incentives to contribute to the eradication effort and may pose a challenge if the initiative does not appear to provide direct benefits to the donor(s) and if fundraising activities will consequently need to appeal to altruistic ideals.

In the past, financing of global and regional public goods occurred primarily through four channels: public sources, private sources, payments by users and beneficiaries, and partnerships (Ferroni and Modi 2002). Principal sources of public financing include developing country governments, donor countries, and multilateral development banks through grants or loans. The opportunity to pursue alternative financing, which may result from developing an EIC that financial leaders can evaluate, represents an important innovation for eradication initiatives. Recognizing that current eradication efforts depend on a pay-as-you-go financial model and that this may lead to resource constraints and nonoptimal operational decisions that ultimately delay eradication and increase overall costs (Duintjer Tebbens and Thompson 2009), we discussed the concept of exploring alternative financing mechanisms for eradication.

In contrast with the current view, we need to conceptualize eradication initiatives as major public health projects (Thompson and Duintjer Tebbens 2008b) that yield public goods with intergenerational benefits. Thus, we should consider eradication in the same manner as major capital investments, and finance them using similar models. Take, for example, the potential issuance of "eradication bonds," which would serve to finance eradication initiatives. Such bonds provide time-limited support and allow sharing the benefits and costs of eradication initiatives with future generations, similar to the concept of the GAVI International Finance Facility for Immunization (IFFIm) (GAVI Alliance 2010c). Eradication bonds may offer the opportunity to front-load funds and provide a steady stream of resources for program implementation, to be repaid with funds intended for similar future development projects. From an ethical standpoint, the eradication bond concept provides a just and fair distribution of benefits and burdens; since future generations will benefit from the eradication of disease, they can in fairness contribute to repayment of the debt.

Special Drawing Rights and the sale of International Monetary Fund gold reserves could provide additional sources of innovative financing opportunities (IMF 2010). Since eradication initiatives may wish to create flexible mechanisms to raise funds quickly, we also discussed the concept of establishing a special-purpose global lottery with tax-free earnings. This could potentially play an important role in financing the end stage of eradication, but might also prove useful in meeting unanticipated funding needs earlier in the program. For eradication initiatives with limited geographical areas, the eradication initiative should engage relevant regional, international financial institutions (e.g., the Asian Development Bank, African Development Bank) to explore strategies to meet funding needs. Finally, we discussed the need to develop potential strategies to engage high net worth individuals, NGOs, and private foundations who might play an important role by providing voluntary contributions.

We emphasize that many opportunities exist to learn from the experiences of prior eradication initiatives, with respect to estimating required financial needs and to including the provision of finances to address unexpected issues. Operational research must be funded and conducted to inform programmatic decisions and make appropriate course corrections, so as to permit identification and solution of unexpected issues. In addition, eradication initiative costs may balloon during the final stages of eradication, due to the very high global control and aggressive efforts needed to reach every infected individual.

A financial concept should potentially allow for a smoothing of costs (e.g., conversion of the balloon payment mortgage to a fixed-rate mortgage), greater ability to fund forward (i.e., make funds available when needed), and expectations for financial management and accountability associated with managing borrowed funds. Such an approach differs significantly from the mode currently used for public health effort, and the partnership responsible for future eradication initiatives would need to be empowered to borrow on the behalf of future generations.

Phasing and the Overall Disease Eradication Portfolio

Discussions about eradication may occur for any individual disease at various points in the life cycle of the disease. Thus, the disease life cycle constitutes an integral part of the discussion (Thompson and Duintjer Tebbens, this volume). Efforts to stop an emerging disease prior to allowing it to become established (e.g., SARS) should proceed based on the available and evolving data about the emerging disease. The EIC should consider the determinants of virulence and host tropism as well as the wide uncertainty bounds in any modeling used to assess the threat. For malaria, some countries (e.g., those on the edges of endemic areas) continue to make significant progress toward achieving national elimination. The achievements led to discussions about the tools needed to achieve malaria eradication, given the challenges associated with sustaining the current high levels of control, and highlighted the need to develop an EIC for each individual disease.

In the context of discussing multiple diseases, we noted that the current disease eradication portfolio includes two initiatives (i.e., dracunculiasis and polio), which operate on very different geographic scales and require distinct types of interventions. Specifically, as a vaccine-preventable viral disease that can rapidly spread globally, polio differs from the parasitic disease guinea worm, which spreads locally and regionally through contaminated water. Coupling these two existing initiatives provides diversity, which portfolio managers generally seek. Essentially, they exist in parallel, with little to no overlap or synergy between them. In addition, combining disease eradication programs might effectively share resources. Potential candidates include measles, onchocerciasis (river blindness), lymphatic filariasis, or other diseases currently targeted for elimination.

Could potential synergies present cost-sharing opportunities to pursue additional eradication initiatives? Figure 10.1 depicts a timeline for multiple eradication initiatives, where t_0 represents the current point in time. At t_0, eradication initiatives A and B are underway (solid arrows represent the current projected, but uncertain end times). Assuming that the EIC for eradication of disease C supports an eradication goal and financing exists to support this goal, the decision to commit to the eradication of C may occur. Up until that point, C will continue with control, and we emphasize that Figure 10.1 does not include the portfolio of controlled infectious diseases. With respect to evaluating C and

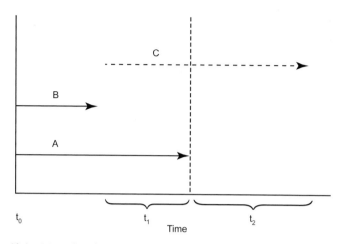

Figure 10.1　Managing the eradication portfolio.

potential synergies with *A* and *B*, the development of a specific analysis that will explicitly consider the synergies may make the combined costs of working on *A* and *C* lower if implemented simultaneously than the costs of completing *A* and *C* independently. With full acknowledgment that *A* and *C* may involve different stakeholders, partnerships, and champions, we suggest the need for explicit characterization of the investment case for disease *C* jointly with *A*, to explore whether opportunities for synergy exist. In this regard, the timing of the launch of *C* could begin anywhere. Figure 10.1 shows the possibility that success of eradication of *B* occurs and launch of the eradication of *C* begins such that *A* and *C* occur simultaneously during the time period t_1, and *C* continues on its own during t_2.

Managing a disease eradication portfolio warrants careful consideration to ensure that resources get used optimally and to avoid eradication efforts "competing" with each other, thus leading to less-than-optimal outcomes (Duintjer Tebbens and Thompson 2009). To counteract the possibility of antagonistic effects (e.g., impacts on existing health systems; see Pate et al., this volume) requires careful consideration of potential antagonistic effects as well as synergies.

In the overall eradication portfolio, numerous criteria related to the decision-making process on the phasing and timing of multiple eradication initiatives should be considered: the nature of interventions, surveillance, scope, staff, costs, social motivation, social and political will, operational issues, and the potential impact on health systems due to codependency on key factors (e.g., two groups potentially competing for resources). A phased approach could make the most sense, because different countries operate on different geographical scales, and phasing efforts may promote continued use and leverage of existing eradication resources or infrastructure, including social and intellectual capital. Bundled activities may permit risks to be shared—a potential that should be carefully scrutinized. If programs link tightly, then issues and challenges that impact one program may spill over to the other program.

In the analysis of the overall eradication portfolio, the process should consider explicitly public perception of eradication efforts and manage public support. Perceptions about one eradication initiative might impact others, such that public perception can act as a significant enabler or barrier for stakeholder engagement and cooperation.

What the Eradication Investment Case Is Not

Clearly, this chapter reflects our aspirations and the promise of an EIC, but it also needs to present what the EIC will not include or achieve. The EIC does not include a financing plan or an implementation plan, focus on country-specific costs and benefits, or make the decision for the world. An EIC should help inform future eradication decisions. However, the actual decision-making process requires weighing multiple attributes, and this depends on values.

We intend that the EIC should provide comprehensive information relevant to the attributes that concern decision makers as they engage in the decision-making process to implement an eradication program. Decision makers are in the best position to make a choice based on their values.

Recommendations

We offer the following recommendations with respect to further development and use of an EIC to support future eradication initatives:

1. Future eradication initiatives should develop an EIC, which we believe will serve to manage expectations more effectively, create opportunities to seek financing and develop better financing plans, and encourage the consideration of eradication initiatives as major projects that provide public goods.
2. All stakeholders should feel empowered to engage in the iterative process used to develop and use EICs. We identified the importance of creating an analytic-deliberative process and recommend the conduct of research that might further define the actual process and the roles of various stakeholders.
3. Recognizing the challenges inherent in integrating large amounts of information into an EIC, efforts should be undertaken to develop specific guidelines for EICs that may help to standardize the process, assist analysts with respect to methodological challenges, and ensure completeness.

4. Additional research should explore the timing, phasing, and portfolio of all eradication efforts and address the joint effects and synergies.
5. Policy makers should identify and research potential options for innovative financing for eradication initiatives, such as eradication bonds.
6. Public health leaders should recognize the challenges associated with managing major projects and learn lessons that may help with respect to managing eradication initiatives.

11

Guidelines for Preparing an Eradication Investment Case

Damian G. Walker and Regina Rabinovich

Abstract

This chapter describes ongoing efforts to develop guidelines for the development of an eradication investment case (EIC). While a single process for the creation or updating of an EIC will likely not exist, three phases of an EIC are proposed (pre-launch, implementation, and completion) and a number of important assumptions associated with the process are highlighted. This chapter updates the list of the "critical elements" of an EIC identified at the Ernst Strüngmann Forum and summarizes a meeting convened afterward to create a template for the EIC guidelines. The intent of the guidelines is to assist analysts with respect to methodological challenges and to ensure completeness. They are an extension of the work accomplished at the Forum and have benefited from additional expertise in the areas of economics and ethics. The final product is envisioned to be practical in nature, going beyond a description of what to do, by describing how to do it with respect to some core methodological issues. This chapter summarizes the work to date and updates the list of the "critical elements" identified at the Forum.

The Process of Preparing an Eradication Investment Case

The term *eradication investment case* (EIC) was conceptualized by Thompson et al. (this volume) as the virtual counterpart of the GAVI Vaccine Investment Case (GAVI Alliance 2004), which is the body of data presented to the GAVI Alliance upon which an evaluation is based and investment commitments are made to finance the introduction of vaccines for low-income, eligible countries. Although decisions for both investment cases require donor and country financing as well as action, there are significant differences. First, while the GAVI Alliance represents the major fund for purchase of vaccines for low-income countries, no such single parallel organization exists for global eradication initiatives. Second, the decision to introduce or scale up a vaccine does not require concerted action from multiple countries, as is critical to an eradication initiative. Third, inherent in an eradication initiative is the need to reevaluate strategies and raise funds late into the program, when disease levels are low or nonexistent, but crucial surveillance and other post-elimination activities must be sustained.

The EIC can thus be conceived as having three phases. In the first *pre-launch phase*, it represents the business plan created with the input of the broad array of funding and implementing partners whose participation is critical to seek funding and cross the line from control to an eradication program. As such, it is a tool that formalizes the ability to analyze the strategies, requirements, risks, and management tools required for success. In the second *implementation phase*, it is transformed into a tactical and financial plan, which must be updated periodically, to address the programmatic and financial challenges that emerge. Ultimately, in the final *completion phase*, it must make a compelling and credible case for completing the task, made particularly challenging at a point when disease levels are extremely low and the disease does not itself represent a national priority based on burden of disease. In the completion phase, financing becomes hostage to donor fatigue, and the progress and costs to the final goal are most challenging.

Given the various ways that eradication initiatives are historically organized and implemented, it is difficult to conceive of a single process for the creation and updating of the EIC. It might be useful, therefore, to consider instead some assumptions regarding the process that emerged from the Forum discussions:

- The decision to create an EIC will have been preceded by a substantive body of work that compels the relevant community to envision global eradication. Thus, the length of time required to compile the EIC must allow for writing the plan, building consensus around implementation strategies, and critical review. Ultimately, however, it will depend on the robustness of the supporting database.
- The role of the champion was recognized as critical for success, but a champion is also clearly biased toward action. Thus, during the pre-launch phase, as the science base is being constructed, the EIC may benefit from being coordinated by a neutral body. However, it must engage the leadership of the community and be "owned" by the relevant experts.
- The systematic construction and evaluation of the EIC can become a powerful tool for the evaluation of competing eradication initiatives. Similarly, it can generate additional thinking around synergies with other disease control and eradication initiatives that leverage human and financial resources.
- It became clear in discussion with leaders of previous initiatives that what is new here is not the creation of a plan for presentation to global policy and decision-making bodies, but rather the attempt to systematize the elements, advance a core methodology, and ensure that appropriate review is conducted.

- Evidence-based external review is critical for credibility and can be achieved through open and blinded review, publication in peer-reviewed literature, and analysis by stakeholders. Some of the key groups capable of evaluating substantively include the technical advisory groups for disease initiatives: the World Health Organization (WHO) expert review, the Carter Center's International Task Force for Disease Eradication, and special commissioned reviews.

- There are a number of potential customers for such an analysis and versions of the final document. These include disease experts, Ministers of Health of affected countries, particularly as embodied by the WHO, regional offices, and advisory groups, and its World Health Assembly; donors (countries, bilaterals) and other funders (philanthropy); civil society and other local implementing partners; and, finally, the people in affected countries who must ultimately be willing to engage in such an endeavor.

As envisioned, the EIC would become the basis for subsequent advocacy, but it does beg the question as to how financing for an eradication initiative can be facilitated. Leadership, technical consensus, and a clear business plan are all necessary components, but would ideally align against the ability to raise funds of the magnitude required for such a program. The Forum considered some innovative approaches to accomplishing this (Thompson et al., this volume), and if such a mechanism were to be created, we believe its effectiveness would be facilitated by having a clearly laid out, reviewed and accepted EIC.

The Boston Meeting

At the Forum, Thompson et al. (this volume) recommended that "efforts should be undertaken to develop specific guidelines for EICs that may help to standardize the process, assist analysts with respect to methodological challenges, and ensure completeness." With the goal of creating a template for the EIC, a subsequent meeting was convened in Boston, Massachusetts, on December 9–10, 2010, to begin the process of standardizing the methodology required to prepare an EIC in support of the decision-making process involved in launching an eradication initiative. The final product, *Guidelines for Preparing an Eradication Investment Case*, is envisioned to be a practical document that describes what needs to be done and, in a few instances, delineates how to do it (e.g., discounting future benefits). To ensure that the development of the EIC guidelines met the expectations expressed at the Forum, additional expertise was brought into the process (Box 11.1). To structure the meeting, we began with the provisional list of critical elements necessary for an EIC identified by Thompson et al. (this volume). Participants were assigned a selection of these elements to develop in advance of the Boston meeting. Small groups were

---

Box 11.1   List of participants to the EIC methodology workshop held in Boston, MA, December 9–10, 2010.

Kimberly Thompson*   Kid Risk, Boston, MA, U.S.A. (Moderator)

Damian Walker*   BMGF, Seattle, WA, U.S.A. (Rapporteur)

Debbie Atherly   PATH, Seattle, WA, U.S.A.

David Bishai   Johns Hopkins School of Public Health, Baltimore, MD, U.S.A.

Lesong Conteh*   Imperial College, London, U.K.

Radboud Duintjer Tebbens   Kid Risk, Boston, MA, U.S.A.

Claudia Emerson*   McLaughlin-Rotman Centre for Global Health, Toronto, Canada

Lee Hall*   National Institutes of Health, Bethasda, MD, U.S.A.

Raymond Hutubessy   World Health Organization, Geneva, Switzerland

Julia Lupp   Ernst Strüngmann Forum, Frankfurt, Germany

James Lavery   McLaughlin-Rotman Centre for Global Health, Toronto, Canada

Jacqueline Leslie   Imperial College, London, U.K.

Ann Levin   Independent consultant, Bethesda, MD, U.S.A.

Maria Merritt   Johns Hopkins School of Public Health, Baltimore, MD, U.S.A.

Regina Rabinovich*   BMGF, Seattle, WA, U.S.A.

Fabrizio Tediosi   Centre for Research on Health and Social Care Management, Bocconi University, Milan, Italy

Anna Vassall   London School of Hygiene and Tropical Medicine, London, U.K.

Maya Vijayaraghavan*   Centers for Disease Control and Prevention, Atlanta, U.S.A.

* Member of the discussion group at the Ernst Strüngmann Forum

   Peter Singer, a member of the original discussion group, was unable to
   participate

---

assigned on the basis of each participant's area of expertise, recognizing that all participants were expected to provide feedback on other elements not assigned to them at the meeting.

Participants were sent a copy of the *Guidelines for Preparing Proposals for GAVI/Vaccine Fund Investment*, because they were perceived to be a useful starting point (notwithstanding a number of important differences in the nature of the investment decisions noted above; see also Thompson et al., this volume). In addition, an example of a submitted investment case, *Accelerating the Introduction of Rotavirus Vaccines into GAVI-Eligible Countries* (PATH's Rotavirus Vaccine Program 2006), which had been worked on by Deborah Atherly, one of the participants, was provided. For the sections of the EIC that focus on the economic evaluation of eradication compared to the status quo, the EIC builds on the WHO's guide for standardization of economic evaluations of immunization programs (WHO 2008a) adding to that framework to account specifically for eradication-related issues (e.g., discounting and intergenerational equity, costing the "last mile"). Participants also referred to their own work on eradication (see, e.g., Emerson and Singer 2010; Duintjer Tebbens et al. 2011) as well as recent efforts to examine the technical feasibility of measles

(WHO 2010a) and malaria eradication (e.g., work of the Malaria Eradication Research Agenda and the Malaria Elimination Group). Participants sent drafts of their sections to Damian Walker, in advance of the meeting, so that a first complete draft of the EIC document could be prepared. In Boston, the participants then worked through this document together, discussing in detail each section and sub-section. As a result of these deliberations, the list of critical elements was revised (Box 11.2).

Structure of the EIC Guidelines

The EIC guidelines are structured around the revised list of critical elements (Box 11.2). To provide requisite guidance, each element begins with a brief description of what the section should cover and why. Where appropriate, recommendations will be made to promote standardized methods (e.g., discounting and intergenerational equity, type of modeling). For example, the choice of discount rate is particularly critical when evaluating the cost-effectiveness of an eradication program. Whereas most general guidelines recommend that health effects be presented as both discounted and undiscounted values, in the context of an eradication program, a zero discount rate for health effects would lead to an intractable analysis due to the infinite benefits arising from a successful eradication program. Therefore, a near-zero discount rate for health effects, lower than the rate for costs, could be considered. An alternative approach to recognizing the intergenerational benefits of successful eradication of a disease is to apply a nonconstant discount rate (declining or "slow") when presenting results (Jamison and Jamison 2003). The EIC guidelines will provide guidance on this core methodological issue.

Each section will also be accompanied by a series of questions to ensure that the group developing an EIC for a specific disease addresses each issue in sufficient detail. These questions will also form the basis of a checklist designed to help promote complete submissions and assist external review of submissions. To illustrate this approach, the preliminary text from Section I.4 is presented in Box 11.3. This section addresses the issue of public goods obtainable by eradication.

In general public health represents a *public good* in the sense that the "benefits to one person cannot readily be individuated from those to another" (Faden and Shebaya 2010). In economic parlance, public goods are collective goods (e.g., disease prevention) that resist efficient market allocation because they can be provided for some people only through efforts that will inevitably benefit others ("free riders"). The prospect that free riders will benefit from a public good without assuming the burdens of producing it is likely to reduce the motivational power of self-interest as an incentive to assume those burdens. For this reason, some public goods may be obtainable only through nonmarket actions (Powers and Faden 2006:144–145). Some public goods in the economic

Box 11.2 Revised structure of the EIC Guidelines.

Section I: The Proposed Investment

I.1   Description of the disease and its global health significance
I.2   Characterization of the status quo
I.3   Articulation of a specific plan for achieving eradication,
I.4   Discussion of the public goods obtainable by eradication
I.5   Discussion of the need for cooperation to obtain the public good

Section II: Rationale for Investing

II.1   Documentation of biological and technical feasibility and review of evidence related to proof of concept
II.2   Indications that stakeholders do or do not want eradication
II.3   Projection of burden of disease expected over the time horizon for analysis: status quo vs. the eradication effort
II.4   Anticipated ethical, social, and political challenges and constraints associated with eradication
II.5   Discussion of how the global plan integrates with and strengthens health systems
II.6   Identification of risks associated with eradication
II.7.   Discussion of the "critical" risks over the entire time horizon of the plan, including the post-eradication stage
II.8   Assessment of total costs associated with an eradication plan
II.9   Assessment of health outcomes associated with eradication plan
II.10   Transparent discussion of broader social impacts
II.11   Assessments of cost-effectiveness and benefit-cost
II.12   Discussion of projected impacts on demand and supply of the interventions and the effect on prices and availability
II.13   Discussion of capacity of qualified staff and technical resources
II.14   Discussion of assumptions about post-eradication plans

Section III: Leadership, Management, and Governance

III.1   Discussion of proposed eradication initiative partnerships and the plan for governance
III.2   Establishment of critical milestones and the plan for monitoring, oversight, and evaluation of milestones
III.3   Assessment of diagnostic tools for monitoring
III.4   Discussion of the risk management plan for critical risks
III.4   Discussion of the operational research plan and the proposed strategy for how operational research would be supported
III.5   Discussion of the proposed process for active evaluation of any impacts on health systems

Section IV: References

Box 11.3   Preliminary text to one section of the EIC Guidelines.

Section I.4   Discussion of the Public Goods Obtainable by Eradication

This section should describe why eradication would contribute uniquely to the attainment of public goods. It should thus answer whether eradication is necessary to provide, protect, and promote the public good in question. It should define what economic public goods would be obtained through eradication, and how these benefits can be captured quantitatively. In doing so, it may be helpful to answer the following questions:

- What public goods are already served by the status quo?
- Are there unique public goods that arise from eradication that do not arise from the status quo? What is special/different about zero incidence as compared with status quo
- Are there incremental gains in public goods to which eradication will contribute?
- Are there any failures in the provision, protection, or promotion of public goods that can be remedied, if at all, only by eradication? Addressing this question will require making the case that eradication remedies the failure.
- What is the nature of the economic public goods?

---

sense also contribute to aspects of the *common good* as understood in political philosophy. To serve the common good is to serve the interest held in common by all members of the public in "self-protection or preservation from threats of all kinds to their welfare" (Beauchamp 2007).

The investment case for eradication should focus on its *unique* contributions to public goods. For any eradication candidate, we expect that the status quo already incorporates concerted efforts to promote multiple public goods. For instance, the status quo should already promote public confidence and global security; eradication activities should continue to do so. The relevant question then becomes: How does eradication provide, protect, and promote public goods in ways that the status quo cannot? For purposes of this comparison, the EIC may also consider contributions to public goods that are necessary means to achieving eradication and are unlikely to be pursued otherwise (e.g., international cooperative financing mechanisms). To the extent that these contributions may remain in place post-eradication (based on realistic expectations), can they be obtained *only* as part of the eradication effort?

Conclusions

Although it is unlikely that any one single process can support the creation or updating of an EIC, we propose three general phases:

- A *pre-launch phase* enables an analysis of the strategies, requirements, risks, and management tools required for success. It is the "business plan," developed through the input of a broad array of partners, whose participation is critical in crossing the line from control to an eradication initiative.

- The *implementation phase* transforms the business plan into a tactical and financial plan—one which must be updated periodically to address emerging programmatic and financial challenges.
- The *completion phase* focuses on work necessary to complete the task (e.g., donor fatigue or challenges that result when disease levels are extremely low and the disease does not represent a national priority based on burden).

Efforts are underway to develop guidelines to support this process. These EIC guidelines are intended to assist analysts with respect to methodological challenges and ensure completeness when preparing the EIC. The development and finalization of the guidelines requires, however, its own process of review and revision. Once a final draft has been prepared, it will be subjected to rigorous, open and transparent review.[1] In addition, the guidelines will also be revised in light of feedback received from groups who submit EICs, and over time, as an EIC moves through the phases of pre-launch, implementation, and completion.

As efforts continue to confront the incalculable misery caused by scourges of disease, it is our sincere hope that the EIC will prove to be a useful tool to the many different stakeholders involved. We look forward to seeing the first applications of the guidelines.

---

[1] For current information on the EIC guidelines, see www.eic-guidelines.org

Governance

are structures of human relationships designed to achieve goals through work (Roberts 2004). A *trans-organizational system* is an "organization of organizations able to make decisions and perform tasks on behalf of member organizations, while the member organizations maintain their separate identities and goals" (Roberts 2004). A trans-organizational system bridges specialist identities and accountabilities of member organizations to produce a new knowledge base. The following characteristics are typical of a trans-organizational system (Cummings and Worley 1996):

- They tend to be under-organized.
- Relationships among organizations are loosely coupled.
- Leadership and power are dispersed among autonomous organizations, rather than hierarchically centralized.
- Commitment and membership are tenuous because member organizations attempt to maintain their autonomy while jointly performing.
- Knowledge management is a core function.

Although the concept of a trans-organizational system has been widely utilized for global health initiatives, they are more commonly referred to as partnerships, alliances, or coalitions.

The concept of the *megacommunity* is a valuable tool for eradication initiatives. Defined as "the means in which organizations and people deliberately join together around a compelling issue of mutual importance, following a set of practices and principles that make it easier for them to achieve results" (Gerencser et al. 2008), it is useful in thinking through the structure, management, and evolving needs of an eradication initiative. Establishing a megacommunity (Figure 12.1) requires a fundamental shift in thinking as work must be organized across multisector and multinational boundaries.

Eradication initiatives require high levels of coordination, cooperation, and collaboration. Because of the diversity and number of actors in the system, the time required to reach the goal (multidecade), and the volatile global environment in which they operate, eradication initiatives require the development of processes to formalize and support the strategy of working together. In addition, while accountability among the interdependent organizations is highly diffuse, it requires active monitoring and management.

Much can be learned from the private sector. The failure rate of private sector alliances has been estimated to be as high as 70%, with most of this failure attributed to an over-emphasis on defining the plan and minimizing conflict (Hughes and Weiss 2007). Understanding and defining how organizations work together, make decisions, allocate resources and cultivate mutual trust must be identified in the formative stages of an initiative and revisited, at a minimum, on an annual basis. To develop the good working relationships within an alliance, Hughes and Weiss (2007) identify four key areas that can be applied to an eradication initiative:

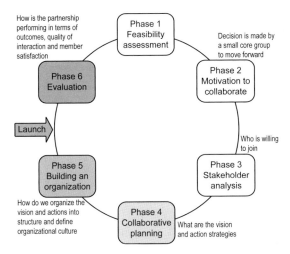

Figure 12.1   Process of establishing a megacommunity.

1. Peg metrics to progress: Augment "ends" metrics with "means" metrics to assess factors that affect the alliance's performance (e.g., information sharing and new idea development).
2. Leverage differences: The fundamental principle of organizing diverse actors around a complex problem is to create value in the alliance; however, those differences may also result in conflict. Instead of driving conflict underground and forcing consensus, leverage those differences to innovate.
3. Encourage collaboration: When a problem surfaces, replace finger-pointing with an analysis of how all parties contributed to it and derive creative solutions to solve it.
4. Manage internal stakeholders: Alliances depend on cooperation and collaboration among leaders of those organizations as well as employees and associates. Everyone needs to have a clear understanding of the goals and their organization's role in achieving success.

Organizational arrangements and structures help create a shared understanding around governance options to structure and manage the work. Ultimately, structural arrangements need to reduce bureaucracy and simplify work toward a common goal (Nohria et al. 2003).

The decision-making process inherent in a trans-organizational system is based on information of various kinds that flows into the system. Current technology enables rapid communication between vast numbers of people in a highly decentralized, informal way. It affects the way individuals collaborate and conduct work, and has been credited with the creation of "new transnational communities of people, who without ever seeing each other in the flesh, are in communion because they are in communication" (Drucker 2001).

Social science and management research can inform an eradication initiative, as it seeks to align and manage the diverse actors involved and mobilize scarce resources. To examine organizational options, five areas of management theory are reviewed: institutional mapping, leadership and skills, nontraditional decision-making processes, organizational culture, and the mobilization and alignment of financial resources. This perspective is applied to eradication initiatives and used to inform resource mobilization and aid frameworks.

Institutional Mapping: Understanding the Dynamic Ecosystem of Actors

Unless commitment is made, there are only promises and hopes; but no plans.
—Peter Drucker

At the outset of an eradication initiative, an analysis of the actors (agencies, stakeholders, individuals, and groups) involved needs to be conducted, as diverse actors influence the way work is organized, distributed, and measured and how results are communicated. This analysis needs to be reviewed periodically to include all of the actors that may influence work over time. In management, *environmental scanning* is the term used to refer to the process of monitoring the environment on an ongoing basis (Roberts 2004; Fahey et al. 1981). Anyone who might implement the vision and strategy or who could block implementation should be included (Kotter 2001). Figure 12.2 illustrates a landscape analysis for an eradication initiative.

After scanning, actors should be characterized into five broad categories (Ibarra and Suesse 1997):

1. Allies share a high level of agreement and trust and often engage in a reciprocal relationship.
2. Opponents share high levels of trust, but agreement is low, and strength and vision are challenged in a trustworthy atmosphere.
3. Bedfellows are aligned with the stated objectives but do not always give the entire story; thus, boundaries must be set.
4. Fence sitters refuse to take a stand so that risk and uncertainty dominate.
5. Adversaries result when attempts at negotiation agreement and trust fail.

Actors (organizations, individuals) may migrate from one category to another during the course of an eradication initiative. For example, during the formative stage, funders may be classified as an opponent because they may need to be persuaded as to the cost-effectiveness of the investment. After classification, an engagement strategy is required for each category—one that is targeted to the vital interests of the principal actors. Engagement strategies assist leaders as they prioritize outreach efforts. Periodic monitoring of relationships offers valuable information on the efficacy of an initiative and can alert leaders to potential problems. Tools, such as annual surveys disseminated to key

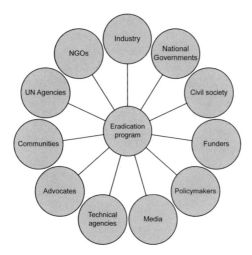

Figure 12.2   Landscape analysis of actors.

stakeholders at various levels of their organizations, can provide comprehensive feedback to managers and enable a strategy to adapt.

Next, a feasibility assessment should be conducted to analyze each stakeholder's level of interest and willingness to commit time and resources to the goal. Data can be collected through surveys, interviews, informal meetings, or broad stakeholder meetings focused around the following questions (Roberts 2004):

- Are other organizations likely to be concerned with this problem as well (i.e., can the base of stakeholders be expanded)?
- Is there willingness to commit time and resources to the work involved on a long-term basis? What assets and capabilities might be exchanged in the partnership? What might each organization provide and expect to receive?
- What kind of work would the group (i.e., stakeholder) undertake?
- What kind of commitment would a core group need to make to get the initiative running?
- What risks are involved (e.g., to a group's reputation, financial)?
- What other benefits might this partnership bring to the organization, to the communities, as well as to the global health sector?
- Is there a strong potential for a partnership that will further a stakeholder's mission and serve its constituency better?

This will lead to an understanding of the strengths and weaknesses involved in the collective assets available to launch the eradication initiative.

The next task is to develop the organizing principles and accountability structures of the initiative within the context of the broader external environment. One classic planning tool is the SWOT analysis (Strengths, Weaknesses,

Opportunities and Threats), which is designed to assess external (opportunities, threats) and internal (strengths, weaknesses) challenges. By assisting leaders in the identification of assets and barriers, SWOT functions like a stakeholder analysis. It can be used to shape the strategy and prioritization of resources and can provide valuable information to the risk management plan.

Because an eradication initiative operates in a highly dynamic environment, both positive and negative trends must be monitored. For this, routine analysis of three key components within the external environment is recommended (Andreasen and Kotler 2008):

1. Public environment: local publics such as disease endemic communities, activists, general public (in both donor and disease endemic countries), media, and regulatory agencies.
2. Competitive environment: groups and organizations that compete for attention, resources, and loyalty.
3. Macroenvironment: large-scale fundamental forces that shape opportunities and pose threats; these forces largely represent the "uncontrollables" and may include demographic, economic, technological, political, and social forces.

Leadership and Skills Mix

> The good leader is he who the people revere. The great
> leader is he who people say, "We did it ourselves."
> —Lao Tzu

Effective leadership in an eradication initiative involves a blend of skills: expertise in public health, leadership, management, finance, marketing, communications, fundraising, policy, supply chain management, regulatory issues, global markets, and international development. Historically, public health experts have taken the lead in global health partnerships. However, future eradication initiatives would benefit from shared leadership between health experts and generalists. The experience that generalists have in negotiating dynamic political, social, and business environments could lessen the inherent risk in complex operational and environmental conditions.

In any collaboration, the manner by which organizations and actors organize around the work ultimately determines effectiveness. Leadership focuses the attention on the task and deploys the necessary resources for execution. It aligns participating organizations around vital interests and ensures that core values are adopted by stakeholders. It focuses on a cogent strategy and decisions, not structure.

Leaders prepare organizations for change and help them adapt (Kotter 2001). They establish a vision and anchor that vision into the organization by inspiring collective and authentic action (Collins 2001). Leaders look for patterns, cultivate interest, and set direction. Effective leaders are masters at motivation. They utilize an individual's need for achievement, affirmation, and affiliation while cultivating a deep sense of purpose (Cialdini 2001).

In a megacommunity, shared leadership is imperative. Each individual leader needs to understand how their leadership style affects the broader group and align their capabilities accordingly with their peer's strengths. Six basic types of leadership styles have been identified (Goleman 2000):

1. A coercive leader demands immediate compliance and emphasizes achievement, initiative, and self-control.
2. An authoritative leader mobilizes people around a vision and uses self-confidence, empathy, and power to catalyze change.
3. An affiliative leader creates harmony, builds emotional bonds, and emphasizes empathy, relationships, and communication.
4. A democratic leader forges consensus through participation and relies on collaboration, team leadership, and communication.
5. A pacesetter sets high standards for performance through conscientiousness, initiative, and a drive to achieve.
6. A coach develops people through empathy and self-awareness.

A mix of leadership styles and skills ensures a diversity of experience and may help to sustain an eradication initiative through difficult stages. Since individual leaders may leave at different points in time, however, successors need to complement the skills of the remaining co-leaders.

Various combinations of leadership styles are required at different stages of an eradication initiative (Table 12.1). At the formative stage, authoritative and democratic styles may be optimal to achieve buy-in and motivate people to

Table 12.1 Combination of leadership styles during the different phases of an eradication initiative.

Formative Stages	
Authoritative	*Democratic*
• Mobilizes toward vision	• Forges consensus
• Catalyzes change	• Relies on collaboration
	• Communication and team leadership

Scaling Up	
Affiliative	*Coaching*
• Creates harmony	• Develops people
• Empathy	• Develops empathy and self-awareness
• Relationships and communication	

Final Mile	
Pacesetting	*Coercive*
• Sets high standards for performance	• Demands immediate compliance
• Drive to achieve	• Emphasizes achievement

action. During the final mile, coercive and pacesetting leadership styles might be more effective to maintain momentum in the face of lagging political or societal interest. Deploying the right leadership style to respond to the changing needs of an eradication initiative and the broader global environment is necessary.

Building an effective leadership team requires an assessment of individuals' leadership styles during the formative stage. This enables individual strengths to be identified and creates a shared understanding of preferences in leadership styles. The tendency to bring in like-minded individuals should be avoided. Miles and Watkins (2007) offer ideas on how leaders can complement one another:

- Task complementarity: leaders divide management and responsibility into coherent blocks of tasks.
- Expertise complementarity: resulting differences lead to formation of teams.
- Cognitive complementarity: differences in how individuals process information; some leaders are better at conceptualizing while others are better at tactics and execution.
- Role complementarity: one or more leaders provide the "pull" through rewards and inspiration while others provide the "push" through disciplined goal setting and sanctions.

To rally support around an initiative, leaders must possess a high degree of emotional intelligence (i.e., self-awareness, self-regulation, motivation, empathy and social skill; Goleman 1995). Conflict can easily arise and create factions or opposing agendas. Thus, leaders must be able to anticipate and understand the viewpoints of partners, and navigate the group to shared goals.

The single most defining feature of an effective leader is a personal motivation. Outstanding leaders continually raise the performance bar and use creativity and a seemingly endless supply of energy to maintain momentum. The greatest challenge to leadership, however, is to facilitate accountability in the multicultural, dynamic, and nonhierarchal structure of any eradication initiative. Understanding how to persuade and motivate effectively within the context of influencing decision making is a crucial leadership skill in any eradication initiative (Williams and Miller 2002).

Nontraditional Decision-making Processes: Power and Persuasion

> Character may almost be called the most effective means of persuasion.
> —Aristotle

In trans-organizational systems, the construction of an organizational chart to articulate where authority lies within the organization is frequently overemphasized. Although important, this step often fails to capture the diffuse and interrelated decision-making process involved in an eradication initiative. Consent, which is a voluntary process, as well as various forms of informal and other nonlegally binding arrangements are required to achieve eradication. However, consent alone cannot drive accountability in the system. Governments, for example, often fail to follow through on pledges made in a World Health Assembly resolution or at the G8 level (McCurry 2008). Understanding how to persuade and motivate within the context of influencing decision making is a crucial leadership skill in an eradication initiative (Williams and Miller 2002). Social capital offers an additional resource and source of soft power in garnering the necessary political will and securing resources.

Eradication initiatives rely on flexibility and agility to respond to the environment in which they operate (social, political, biological). Performance is enhanced when the ability of the interconnected organizations to execute key decisions more effectively is collectively improved (Blenko et al. 2010). Conducting a decision audit helps leaders understand where power and influence are required to achieve alignment and sustain commitment. The following steps are needed to create a decision audit:

1. Identify key decisions to be undertaken.
2. Determine where those decisions should happen.
3. Organize the macrostructure around sources of value.
4. Determine which level of authority is needed by decision makers.
5. Align other elements of the organizational system (e.g., incentives, information flow and processes) with those related to decisionmaking.
6. Help partners develop skills and behaviors necessary to execute high-quality decisions quickly.

Within the framework of an eradication initiative, a decision audit begins with the individual:

- What motivates the individual to accept the intervention, such as a vaccine?
- What factors are associated with the individual's decision to participate?
- What decisions are taken at the local, regional, or national level that facilitate or impede successful execution?
- Who decides, who enables, who has the power to block decisions?

Expanding this exercise to the regional and global level informs strategies designed to support advocacy, policy development, social mobilization, resource mobilization, and various other activities. Decision making, therefore, is not a simple, discrete event, but rather a stream of decisions and choices. One of the benefits of conducting a decision audit is that it scrutinizes the motives behind why a decision was taken, or not taken, and uses this information to persuade the decision maker in a direction that aligns with the goal of the initiative.

Ultimately, a successful eradication initiative results from the sum of the decisions that actors make and execute.

Understanding the decisions which must be taken is only the first step in mapping where accountability needs to exist in the system. Mapping reveals where accountability structures are diffuse and hard to manage, particularly in a system of interdependent actors. Much can be learned from the malaria initiative, where low utilization of insecticide-treated bed nets by individuals in malaria endemic regions jeopardized efforts to eliminate the disease (Ahorlu et al. 1997). Who should be held accountable for this breakdown in the system?

Within the context of management theory, *accountability* is defined as "the means managers are held responsible for carrying out a defined set of duties or tasks, and for conforming with the rules and standards applicable to their posts" (OECD 1998). Within a megacommunity, traditional or hierarchical accountability mechanisms cannot be used to manage the work of interdependent actors; accountability structures must be decentralized between actors and organizations so that performance can be enhanced throughout the entire system. Performance and financial management tools (e.g., dashboards and balanced scorecards) can measure and monitor the progress of various aspects of an initiative and assist in identifying where accountability structures should be enhanced by traditional incentive mechanisms. Failure to achieve results does not necessarily induce accountability from those who are responsible for failing to adopt mitigation strategies or improve performance. If the agreement to collaborate is based on consent or nonlegally binding terms, then traditional, remedial measures will not work. Understanding the complexity in the system of stakeholders as it relates to accountability is a precursor to developing mechanisms that are more effective in sustaining motivation and enhancing collaboration.

Accountability without power can derail a partnership, and research has shown that organizational powerlessness can corrupt (Kanter 1979). Defined as the ability to mobilize resources to get things done, *power* is rooted in the ability to control resources, information, and support necessary to perform a task (Kanter 1979). Power is best utilized when it provides access to resources and information; this enables individuals to act quickly, accomplish more, and give more resources and information to others. Thus, power can be an effective catalyst to manage work efficiently. By contrast, *powerlessness* tends to breed bossiness rather than true leadership; it can create ineffective, petty, dictatorial, and rules-minded managerial styles (Kanter 1979). In an eradication initiative, careful assessment of where accountability exists without the necessary power can help expose risks and improve outcomes by enabling those stakeholders with the necessary power and resources to carry out their work.

The paradigm of high accountability with insufficient power can be illustrated in the relationship between donor countries and national governments (recipients of aid) involved in global health programs. Much has been written about the ineffectiveness of top-down approaches to aid deployment, leading to a shift toward country-led initiatives, donor harmonization, and managing aid for results (OECD 2005). Developing countries are often put in the position of accepting aid according to the terms, plans, and strategies developed by donor governments, contractors, and NGOs. This, in turn, can lead to suboptimal results, because the flexibility required to implement these programs locally was not properly considered. Donor countries, in return, implement performance-based financing, and national governments are left with little choice but to check boxes and comply with ever tighter conditions.

A better approach would be to include developing country health officials in the design and planning of any new health initiative from the outset. This way, issues such as the impact on health systems, integration with other national health initiatives and plans, supply chain and logistics, regulatory considerations and management capacity can be assessed and factored into design and funding arrangements. Consultation can be formal or informal and can be conducted via surveys, interviews, or convening regional meetings. When people are asked for their input, when they know they have been heard and mutual trust has been established, they are more committed to a program. If its results are translated into the design, consultation can empower and ultimately lead to increased accountability and motivation. By empowering others, a leader does not decrease his/her power but may actually increase it (Kanter 1979).

Organizational Culture

> Always bear in mind that your own resolution
> to succeed is more important than any other.
> —Abraham Lincoln

Organizational culture is an emerging concept in the field of management theory. It is a fundamental driver of what an organization sets as its mission, objective, and goals, and what will be expected of those who work to achieve them (Andreasen and Kotler 2008). Organizational culture often refers to the shared beliefs, values, and norms that represent the character of an organization by (a) conveying a sense of identity for organizational members, (b) facilitating the generation of commitment to something larger than self, (c) enhancing social system stability, and serving as a sense-making device to guide and shape behavior (Panda and Gupta 2001).

In megacommunities, organizational culture can be defined as the overarching principles and values that create the foundation of the collaborative effort among various organizations and stakeholders. In the formative stage, it is important to identify the core values and guiding principles that will guide the work and clarify what various stakeholders' roles and responsibilities will be to uphold the principles. Core values improve accountability among stakeholders by becoming the galvanizing force that holds the initiative together.

In an eradication initiative, shared purpose and a convergence around vital interests stem from the deeply held belief that disease eradication is a global public good. Without this core value at the heart of an initiative, it is virtually impossible to garner the political and societal buy-in to sustain the effort over the life of the program. Core values, shared beliefs, and guiding principles should be publically available (e.g., as a central component on partners' websites), stated clearly throughout strategic plans, and reinforced in all communication materials. As ambassadors of the organizational culture, leaders must reinforce core values to maintain motivation and focus among their diverse set of stakeholders.

To boost collaboration and establish trust-building processes in support of the loose accountability structures among stakeholders, the guiding principles of future eradication initiatives should include:

- shared beliefs around purpose,
- requirement for shared leadership,
- fostering a culture of inclusion and sense of belonging and ownership.
- a need for flexibility to adapt to a complex and rapidly changing internal and external environment,
- embracing failure and encouraging risk taking as a fundamental component of learning and improved performance,
- encouraging openness and transparency,
- embracing dynamic tension and conflict as a means to innovate,
- promoting diversity as a driver of value.

Establishing guiding principles helps stakeholders develop a common language, supports communication, and promotes critical thinking and problem solving (Gerencser et al. 2008). It also assists leaders in establishing and managing expectations so as to avoid unnecessary setbacks. The fundamental belief that change and conflict are inherent in the system, as well as the key drivers of innovation and improved performance, is crucial. Historically, too much emphasis has been placed on achieving consensus. In a megacommunity, consensus can lead to "groupthink." Groupthink occurs when a group makes faulty decisions because group pressures lead to a deterioration of mental efficiency, reality testing, and moral judgment. Organizations affected by groupthink ignore alternatives and tend to take irrational actions that dehumanize other groups. A group is especially vulnerable to groupthink when its members are similar in background, when the group is insulated from outside opinions, and when there are no clear rules for decision making (Janis 1982).

To protect against groupthink, Janis (1982) suggests adopting some of the following measures:

- The leader should assign the role of critical evaluator to each member.
- The leader should avoid stating preferences and expectations at the outset.

- One or more experts should be invited to each meeting on a staggered basis. The outside experts should be encouraged to challenge views of the members.
- At least one articulate and knowledgeable member should be given the role of devil's advocate (to question assumptions and plans).

Leaders within a megacommunity need to understand that many decisions are made under conditions of uncertainty. Fostering a culture that challenges one another will create a greater range of options and ultimately enable the group to make better decisions (Eisenhardt et al. 1997). Maintaining a sense of humor, utilizing empathy, focusing on issues and not personalities, and establishing equity in the process enables leaders to use conflict to improve performance (Eisenhardt et al. 1997).

Core values, guiding principles, and a shared purpose are the main drivers of motivation and improved performance among a diverse group of stakeholders. Over time, and if properly managed by leaders, organizational culture can become the bedrock of the initiative, by providing resilience to overcome the inevitable challenges and setbacks that are inherent in an eradication initiative.

Mobilizing and Aligning Financial Resources

Opportunities multiply as they are seized.—Sun Tzu

To ensure long-term success in an eradication initiative, it is necessary to understand how funding flows are coordinated and aligned. Megacommunities are uniquely positioned to leverage funds from their own constituents, civil society groups, corporations, and governments and can amass incredible political and societal support. The challenge, however, is to create incentives that will enhance collaboration among stakeholders and attract resources. It may be easy to gain buy-in around the goal of eradication, but it can be much harder to exact agreement on the sharing of scarce resources. Here, the concept of *co-opetition* may be helpful. First coined by Rockwell Hunt (1937), co-opetition occurs when organizations work together to achieve a specific goal, where one organization does not have a competitive advantage over another, and where all share in common costs and receive greater benefits (resources) because of the collaboration. If a collective effort is successful, all parties should benefit.

To understand how funds flow from the global to local level, it is necessary to analyze how health programs are funded at the national, regional, and global levels. Thereafter, accountability structures designed to attract funding from a diverse group of donors need to be mapped. The mechanisms by which programs are supported and funds are raised and disbursed as well as the similarity among funding requirements between donors have important implications for the efficient and effective use of resources at the national level.

One of the tensions between donors and recipients is the need to balance donor priorities with the requirements of the program on the ground. This needs to be taken into account early in the initiative, so that monitoring and evaluation frameworks can support donor outreach and harmonization efforts. Knowing when to decline donor support must also be defined; for example, when donors are unwilling to align their resources in ways that are beneficial, or at least not disruptive, to ongoing efforts.

After funding flows have been identified and buy-in from key stakeholders has been achieved, fundraising activities can be scaled-up.

Resource Mobilization

The Global Fund to Fight AIDS, Tuberculosis and Malaria (Global Fund) and the Global Alliance for Vaccines and Immunization (GAVI) are the two largest organizations that currently disperse health funding. Their funds, however, are restricted to a core set of diseases or interventions; neither is able, for example, to support guinea worm or lymphatic filariasis initiatives. Efficient use of scarce resources requires well-coordinated work and a clear-cut strategy, otherwise funding can become a contentious and divisive issue in an eradication initiative.

As new treatments and therapeutics are approved for funding, funders come under increasing pressure to provide more resources. The introduction of new vaccines, pediatric malaria formulations, and new treatment kits to prevent vertical transmission of HIV from mother to child represent just a few of the contributing factors to the rising annual costs of GAVI and the Global Fund. Compounding this problem, their leadership has acknowledged that slow disbursement of funds poses an ongoing and growing challenge for countries that need a reliable flow of resources to support their programs. Countries struggle to find and maintain the required human resource support to comply with the monitoring and reporting requirements of the Global Fund. For some countries, this is reported to be complicated and results are inconsistent (Oomman et al. 2007).

Mandated funding has raised the debate about whether the Global Fund should expand its program beyond AIDS, tuberculosis, and malaria. Many countries lack comprehensive funding for health, and thus there is a need to strengthen health systems. More recently, this debate has expanded to include maternal and child health. While an expanded mandate may help countries implement more comprehensive and effective public health programs, it generates pressures on funding during a time of waning political support and strapped financing. The current financial crisis poses a threat to the long-term viability of a growing annual, multibillion dollar fund. In the absence of a new global eradication fund, novel financing mechanisms or ways of coordinating funding flow will be required.

Sustainable sources of funding can be derived by leveraging economic growth in emerging markets as well as in regions where natural resources attract significant levels of foreign direct investment. McKinsey (2010) reports that the "rate of return on foreign investment is higher in Africa than in any other developing region...Real GDP rose by 4.9% a year from 2000 through 2008, more than twice its pace in the 1980s and 1990s. Telecommunications, banking, and retailing are flourishing. Construction is booming. Private-investment inflows are surging." In addition, Africa is rich in natural resources, with more than 60% of the world's uncultivated, arable land (McKinsey 2010). A growing global demand for resources such as food, water, and energy place Africa in the middle of what has become a final resource grab for the world's biggest economies, including India and China (World Economic Forum 2009). Given the availability of natural resources and real GDP growth in Africa, as well as sustained levels of growth in Asia and Latin America, is there an opportunity for the global community to work with national leaders to increase the percentage of GDP and foreign direct investment for global health programs? Reliance on the G8 governments to maintain multibillion dollar commitments in support of global health priorities, when these economies are growing more slowly, warrants a broader discussion.

Conclusion

> You can't depend on your eyes when your imagination is out of focus.
> —Mark Twain

Eradication initiatives require greater coordination, cooperation, and collaboration than traditional organizations because of the independence, diversity, and number of actors involved and the extended timeframes needed for results. Good governance requires institutional mapping, leadership and skills, non-traditional decision-making processes, organizational culture, and the mobilization and alignment of financial resources. At the outset of an eradication initiative:

- An environmental scan of the diverse actors should be conducted to determine how work is organized, distributed, and measured, and how results are communicated.
- A feasibility assessment should be undertaken to analyze each stakeholder's level of interest and willingness to commit to the goal.
- Organizing principles and accountability structures should be developed within the context of the broader external environment.
- Developing country health officials should be involved in the design and planning of the initiative.
- Core values and guiding principles need to be developed to guide work and clarify stakeholders' roles and responsibilities.

- Funding of health programs at the national, regional, and global levels should be assessed.
- Accountability structures that will attract funding from a diverse group of donors need to be mapped.
- Sustainable sources of funding must be sought.

In addition, leadership needs to be comprised of a diverse mix of actors to ensure expertise and galvanize societal will. Countries need to find new sources of power among their citizens and utilize their input to monitor how well the system is working: from the donor level to local communities. Online communities (both mobile and online platforms) should be used to strengthen local communities' ability to collaborate and share best practices.

Interventions, diagnostics, technology, and advances in social science and management theory suggest that the 21st century offers unprecedented opportunities to solve some of the world's greatest health challenges. To do this, however, requires more than tools. Novel approaches are needed to engage a broad set of actors.

Acknowledgments

I wish to acknowledge global health leaders who demonstrate exemplary leadership styles required to guide successful multicultural alliances in the 21st century: Mr. Ray Chambers, United Nations Secretary-General's Special Envoy for Malaria; Dr. Uche Amazigo, Director of the African Programme for Onchocerciasis Control; and Professor David Molyneux, Global Alliance for the Elimination of Lymphatic Filariasis, Liverpool School of Tropical Medicine.

13

Managing Neglected Tropical Disease Partnerships

Andy Wright

Abstract

A key ingredient for success of eradication and elimination initiatives is the formation of an effective partnership among all participating parties. This chapter examines the mechanisms required to manage the partnerships and the delivery of the interventions needed to achieve the eradication and/or elimination goals. Such mechanisms include technical and programmatic leadership; implementation guidelines; supply of diagnostics, drugs, or vaccines; technical and programmatic review; monitoring of progress; evaluation of impact, budgeting and cost management; management of data; safety monitoring and reporting; and inventory management and distribution of drugs and vaccines.

Introduction

The formation of an effective partnership among all participating parties is a key ingredient for success of eradication and elimination initiatives. The concept of partnerships was discussed at an expert colloquium held at the Carter Center (Dentzer 2008), at which Tachi Yamada, from the Bill & Melinda Gates Foundation, stated: "The largest success of the past decade has been the formation of partnerships between private industry, between government, between affected nations and not-for-profit organizations such as ours" (Dentzer 2008:2).

GlaxoSmithKline has participated for more than a decade in the global partnership to eliminate lymphatic filariasis (LF), donating albendazole to reach several hundreds of millions of people in 50 countries. This chapter builds on the GlaxoSmithKline experience and examines the principles of managing a neglected tropical disease (NTD) elimination initiative in partnership with multiple countries to achieve a common goal.

Background

Effective partnerships are essential for successful eradication and elimination initiatives and may involve:

- national governments of individual countries, as represented by the ministries of health, education, finance, and transportation;
- United Nations organizations (WHO, World Bank, and others);
- international donors (bilateral agencies, foundations, and private individuals);
- the pharmaceutical industry, which contributes financial donations and supplies drugs and vaccines;
- nongovernmental organizations (NGOs), which focus on implementation and patient care;
- civil society (patient care); and
- research institutions and universities, which supply scientific and programmatic support.

Each of these diverse partners brings unique strengths and capabilities to bear on the global challenge of disease elimination or eradication. Every effort should be made to ensure those strengths are used optimally.

Published reviews describing the achievements of the partnerships and the lessons that have subsequently been learned are available for onchocerciasis (Thylfors et al. 2008) and leprosy (Braber 2004).

Mechanisms Needed to Implement the Partnerships

To achieve the goals of elimination, a range of mechanisms are required for both the partnerships and the initiatives: a governance structure and forum, defined roles and responsibilities for each partner, shared strategic plan, advocacy and fund raising, and coordination and communication. These are discussed elsewhere and will thus not be repeated here (see, e.g., Stoever, this volume). For a partnership and NTD program to operate effectively, however, specific mechanisms are needed and will be discussed in turn below:

- lead technical and programmatic authority,
- implementation guidelines,
- diagnostic supply,
- drug or vaccine supply,
- technical and programmatic review,
- monitoring progress,
- evaluation of impact,
- budgeting and cost management,
- data management,

- safety monitoring and reporting, and
- inventory management and distribution.

Lead Technical and Programmatic Authority

Because of the nature of NTD elimination programs, a coordinated approach is required across all countries engaged in the effort. For most of the initiatives listed in Table 13.1, WHO fulfills this role. It establishes guidelines for implementation, monitoring, and evaluation and appoints regional and technical groups to guide program implementation and strategy.

Implementation Guidelines

Each NTD program has published guidelines, specifically developed for county program managers, on how to implement an intervention. For many disease programs, delineation of these guidelines is carried out by the WHO as part of its normative function. For example, for the LF elimination program, WHO published a program manager's manual (WHO 2000a) that sets out the methodology on how to plan and implement the interventions, including:

- mapping disease prevalence,
- baseline surveys,
- training,
- mass drug administration,
- social mobilization,
- midterm evaluations,
- stopping of mass drug administration, and
- surveillance after mass drug administration.

More recently, with the emergence of integrated control of NTDs, WHO has published guidelines on preventive chemotherapy for NTD control (WHO 2006c).

For trachoma, the International Trachoma Initiative (ITI) has published detailed guidelines for the implementation of the comprehensive SAFE strategy

Table 13.1   Current elimination programs that target neglected tropical diseases.

Leprosy	Global Alliance for the Elimination of Leprosy http://www.who.int/lep/partners/en/
Onchocerciasis	Onchocerciasis Elimination Program for the Americas (OEPA) http://www.who.int/blindness/partnerships/onchocerciasis_oepa/en/index.html
Trachoma	International Trachoma Initiative http://www.trachoma.org/core/
Lymphatic filariasis	Global Alliance to Eliminate Lymphatic Filariasis http://www.filariasis.org/

(ITI 2010). This publication complements the guidelines for program managers in trachoma control, which was published by WHO (2006d).

Diagnostic Supply

Diagnostics are used to map the prevalence of disease or to identify individual patients for selective treatment. Typically, diagnostic tests are manufactured by for-profit companies and are not donated. Thus a procurement process, with corresponding funding, is necessary.

Depending on the mapping methodology, the size of the country, and disease prevalence, each individual country may require only a relatively small number of diagnostic tests. Typically, however, manufacturers produce tests in batches, and their minimum batch size may far exceed the needs of any one individual country. Coordination is thus required to aggregate small orders from individual countries into large contracts with suppliers. Furthermore, manufacturers often prefer to work with a central procurement organization rather than many individual countries, as this reduces transaction costs. To enable the manufacturer to plan and allocate a slot in the production schedule, it is crucial to coordinate and aggregate forecasts and agree upon a supply schedule in advance. As country needs are clarified, orders can be gathered and combined into large orders to be placed with the manufacturer. Such coordination also enables more effective price negotiation. In the LF elimination program, this coordination role has been performed by the WHO for the provision of immunochromatography card tests. These tests are produced by Inverness and are either financed by the countries themselves, reimbursing WHO directly, or out of donated funds held by the WHO.

Drug or Vaccine Supply

The provision of quality drugs or vaccines in the necessary quantities requires an application process with appropriate reviews as well as a procurement system to ensure delivery to the country program when needed. Once in the country, an effective way of storing, transporting, and controlling products is also required. To ensure the effective supply of drugs or vaccines, the following mechanisms are required and discussed in turn below:

- application, review, and approval process,
- procurement plan,
- quality assurance and control,
- transport,
- in-country storage and logistics,
- warehouse management and control,
- reporting,
- product recalls, and
- an effective way to handle expired drugs and vaccines.

Applications, Reviews, and Approvals

Whether drugs or vaccines are being donated or purchased, a mechanism is needed to quantify and request or order them. Each donation program has its own application form and process. In the LF elimination program, this process is managed by the WHO and involves a standard application form, which is reviewed by Regional Program Review Groups (R-PRGs). A standard application form is needed to capture all of the relevant information, which in turn enables a review group to make a recommendation on the leadership and management of the program, epidemiological data on treatment areas, implementation strategy, budget and funding, requirement for drugs (including inventory calculation), and delivery details.

Countries prepare elimination plans and submit applications for donated drugs to the R-PRG. In the LF elimination program, the following criteria are used by the R-PRGs to evaluate country submissions:

- Ministerial commitment to the elimination of LF.
- The initial proposal must contain the epidemiological and parasitological data required to begin operations. It must also make provision to expand that data progressively as needed to support the requirements of a national program. A phased approach is generally required for larger countries.
- Potential to integrate with other public health services or programs.
- Presence of a national coordination committee or similar body.
- Clear identification of resource requirements needed to implement the intervention program.
- For applications requesting an expansion of initial operations, evidence must show that the targets for the initial operations are being met, the epidemiological data are available to justify the expansion, and the resources for that expansion are adequate.
- Technical capacity is already present or a clear statement of how such capacity will be created.
- Guaranteed exemption from, or counterpart payments for, fees to cover customs duties, acceptance, and clearance. Evidence of mechanisms in place for appropriate drug handling and warehousing must also be demonstrated.
- A plan to have an impact assessment on transmission on a subset or a sentinel group of the treated population.
- The capacity or adequacy to identify, manage, report, and monitor serious adverse experience with drugs used.
- For reapplications, a progress report must have been received detailing progress achieved in the previous mass drug administration and an accounting of tablets used and remaining in stock.

Once the R-PRG approves an application, its recommendation is passed on to the WHO for procurement.

Since each donation program has its own application form and review process, some countries maintain that there is duplication and unnecessary complexity involved in making multiple applications for different drugs (e.g., albendazole, Mectizan®, Zithromax®, mebendazole, diethylcarbamazine). In response, the Task Force for Global Health is currently working on a design for an integrated application, based on a template NTD plan, which can be applied for all drugs used in the NTD programs. Thus far, the only example of an integrated application form in use is one that was developed by the Mectizan Donation Program for use in applying for Mectizan® and albendazole for the LF and onchocerciasis programs in Africa.

Procurement

The mechanisms for donated and procured drugs and vaccines are very similar: donated products are simply procured at zero cost. For drugs donated via the WHO for the LF elimination program, a purchase order must be issued by the WHO procurement system with details of the quantity required, delivery address, due date, mode of transport, and detailed shipping instructions. On this standard WHO purchase order, the quoted price for donated drugs is zero. By using this system, orders are tracked and processed by the WHO according to their standard system and procedures. This alleviates the need to create a new system.

For procured drugs and vaccines, WHO uses the same system to place purchase orders. An evaluative process may, however, be used to establish the supplier and price of the products.

In cases where other partners purchase drugs or vaccines, they may need to adhere to the procurement system of the organization that houses the donation program. For example, in the schistosomiasis control initiative, praziquantel is purchased from generic manufacturers according to the procurement system used by Imperial College, where the initiative is based.

Quality Assurance and Control

Most donations of drugs or vaccines for eradication or elimination initiatives are made by major research-based pharmaceutical companies: Merck & Co., Inc. (Mectizan®), GlaxoSmithKline (albendazole), Pfizer (Zithromax®), and others. These companies are internationally recognized as suppliers of high-quality medicines and have high-caliber assurance and quality control systems. As such, WHO and most country governments are content to rely on the suppliers quality control systems and do not require additional independent testing. In a few cases, countries request inspections prior to shipment or may conduct independent quality testing on samples once they arrive in country.

For initiatives that use nondonated drugs (e.g., diethylcarbamazine for LF or praziquantel for schistosomiasis), WHO usually seeks procurement from generic pharmaceutical companies. To ensure access to good-quality medicines, WHO operates a prequalification process to certify suppliers for inclusion on an approved supplier list. This is a rigorous process which takes time, technical resources, and funds—all of which WHO often lacks.

When an initiative uses nondonated drugs and operates without using WHO as a procurement agent, procurement is arranged directly with generic suppliers. Purchasing medicines from generic suppliers without a prequalification process does not, however, result in the same level of quality assurance. In addition, since different suppliers may be used each time a drug is procured, the drug itself may be delivered in different forms. This can create potential confusion for the user: the tablets provided may look physically different to ones previously used. To assist in the identification of the various drugs used in NTDs, WHO has published an informative newsletter, "Action Against Worms," which contains photographs of the actual drugs used in an intervention (WHO 2006a).

Transport

Drugs and vaccines need to be transported from the manufacturer to the country that needs them. Different programs use different modes of transport—land, sea, or air—depending on the circumstances of each shipment.

Most of the drugs that are used in disease control programs are manufactured in Europe or Southeast Asia, so the opportunity for land transport to countries is limited. One exception is albendazole, which is manufactured in South Africa by GlaxoSmithKline. Albendazole is able to be transported by land to neighboring Mozambique. However, given the poor state of road networks elsewhere, this delivery option is not readily available to other African countries. For land-locked countries in Africa and Asia, overland transport from the port of entry, which may be in another country, is necessary. This has proved especially challenging in several cases, as the transport route changes from one mode to another (often requiring different freight companies) and crosses national borders. For drugs manufactured in the country where they will be used, land transport is the obvious choice. In India, GlaxoSmithKline is able to deliver albendazole, which is manufactured in country, by road to the LF elimination program.

The cost of shipping drugs via sea freight is typically one-tenth of the cost of shipping by air. Thus, from an economic perspective, transportation by sea is preferred. However, sea freight is slow. It takes weeks (and sometimes months) to cross the oceans, and this time lag poses a challenge when planning to ensure that drugs reach the countries in time for the planned distribution program. For the LF elimination program outside of India, GlaxoSmithKline manufactures albendazole tablets in South Africa. The weight and volume of consignments precludes use of air freight in many cases, and thus 95% of albendazole tablets are shipped by sea freight to minimize costs. Greater lead time and close attention to forecasting and management of purchase orders is required to ensure that the shipping time does not delay a country's program.

Since the use of air transport is prohibitively expensive, it is only appropriate for small quantities or light products of high value. For example, most of the Zithromax® donated by Pfizer is sent by air to speed up delivery. It is also seen as a more secure mode of delivery for a high-value product.

Regardless of the transport mode, all shipments must conform to the storage requirements of the products (i.e., typically temperature and humidity conditions). Fortunately, the drugs used in the current NTD control programs are stable and do not generally require special conditions during transport.

In-Country Storage and Logistics

Once delivered to a country, drugs and vaccines need to be stored in appropriate warehouses. Storage must be secure to prevent theft as well as damage from heat, humidity, and other causes. The products then need to be transported by road to the districts for use. Typically, drugs and vaccines are shipped internationally on pallets, which can easily be moved into warehouses and onto container vehicles using forklifts. However, since the vehicles used to transport the goods further once in a country are often too small to accommodate a pallet, pallets must be dismantled so that the boxes can be loaded onto vehicles by hand. In-country transport can be a challenge due to limited availability of adequate vehicles and the poor state of many roads in developing countries, particularly during rainy seasons. Similarly, there is often a lack of suitable storage facilities at peripheral health centers, so drugs and vaccines must be stored in clinics or other available buildings.

Warehouse Management and Control

Good warehouse management is important to maintain control over the inventory and facilitate appropriate use. One important warehouse principle—first in, first out—is utilized to ensure that the oldest dated products are always used first. This may seem obvious; however, in a recent case from the LF elimination program, a country had stocks of drugs left over from the previous year's distribution program, and these were supplemented by a new delivery for the following year's program. The newly delivered drugs were subsequently used first, thus leaving the older drugs stored in the warehouse past their expiration date.

To address such problems, the International Trachoma Initiative recently published guidelines for the effective management of Zithromax® (ITI 2010). This excellent document covers in detail the necessary steps and procedures that are recommended for the effective management of Zithromax®, including receiving drugs, storage, inventory management, record keeping, managing expiry dates, and disposal of expired drugs and empty containers. The principles and procedures described in these guidelines are equally applicable to drugs used in other disease control programs.

Reporting

It is crucial for countries to report on the progress achieved in a program. Reporting is a vital component for all projects, since it allows progress to be measured against the original plan and for this to be taken into account as the next phase is prepared. For disease control programs, it is important to measure the distribution of drugs or vaccines, compliance, and coverage to evaluate whether the strategy being adopted is working effectively or needs to be refined. Regardless of whether funding is being provided from in-country budgets or external donors, all funders want to know how effectively the investment is being used.

For programs that benefit from donated drugs, reporting is particularly important as donors want to know that the drugs supplied have been used to treat the endemic populations and what quantities remain unused. For the LF elimination program, the template progress report (WHO unpublished) contains a simple table to report the number of people treated and a calculation of the quantity of drugs available at the start, those used, and the quantity that remains. This enables the drugs left over to be taken into account when calculating the requirement for the following year. Experience from the LF elimination program has shown that reporting is often poorly completed. On occasion, the calculations provided were inaccurate or contained missing information, which left open the question of what quantity of drugs remain unused each year. Most likely, this resulted from inconsistencies in record keeping within country, which makes it difficult for the national program manager to know what drugs remain in stock at the district level. Unless addressed, this problem could become acute as NTD programs become more integrated and several different drugs are used for the various diseases.

Product Recalls

Occasionally, due to problems in quality, individual batches of a drug or vaccine may need to be recalled. Fortunately, this happens rarely, and I am unaware of any instance having occurred in the current drug donation programs. If such a problem were to occur, however, the manufacturer would issue a recall notice specifying the batch numbers affected. The manufacturer would know which country/countries the affected batches were shipped to and have an audit trail through to delivery. However, once inside a country, the audit trail and recall process would depend on good record keeping to track where the relevant batches were sent.

Expired Drugs and Vaccines

Unused drugs and vaccines left over from programs may occasionally exceed their expiry date. In such cases, expired drugs need to be destroyed in an approved manner: usually high-temperature incineration. Since many developing world countries lack a suitable incineration capacity, expired drugs or vaccines may need to be returned to the manufacturer to be destroyed. Good record keeping and stock management are essential to enable the expired drugs to be located, gathered, and packaged for export back to the supplier.

In the LF elimination program, there have been a few cases of drugs expiring unused, and these have had to be returned to the supplier to be destroyed in the country where they were manufactured.

Technical and Programmatic Review

Disease control, elimination, and eradication programs need appropriate review and technical oversight. Different programs have established their own structures. For example, the African Program for Onchocerciasis Control has established several levels of governance: the Joint Action Forum enables donors to have oversight of the program and the Mectizan Expert Committee provides technical and programmatic oversight.

For the LF elimination program, WHO provides technical and programmatic oversight. When the LF elimination program was launched, WHO established a Technical Advisory Group (TAG) to make recommendations and report back to the WHO on scientific, safety, and programmatic aspects of the elimination program. TAG was later incorporated into the new Strategic and Technical Advisory Group (STAG), which now provides this oversight function for all NTD programs. In addition, R-PRGs were established by the WHO to:

- Review and provide guidance to countries in the development of their national plans of action for LF elimination.
- Review the implementation and progress of national programs to ensure consistency with the regional and global strategies and targets, and to make recommendations to WHO regional focal points on the subsequent requests for up-scaling of programs in subsequent years.
- Provide technical guidance in the implementation of the TAG recommendations when relevant for the member countries of the region.
- Identify operational research issues that arise when programs are in the region and refer these issues to the relevant research institutions of the region and WHO.
- Advise the WHO on matters related to verifying the interruption of transmission of LF in countries of the region.

- Advocate and support the member countries in seeking political commitments from governments and Ministries of Health for the elimination of LF.

These R-PRGs have proved very effective in reviewing progress by the countries, approving applications for donated drugs, and supporting countries as they resolve issues that affect their programs.

Monitoring Progress

The basic strategy behind programs to eliminate or eradicate a disease is to implement an intervention (typically, but not exclusively drug or vaccine treatment) that will bring the transmission of the disease below a specified threshold. Once this has been achieved, the interventions can be stopped and the disease should not reemerge. Program interventions need to be monitored closely to ensure that the treatment strategy is being implemented effectively (particularly the coverage achieved). Once the required number of treatment rounds has been completed, a thorough evaluation of the impact that the program has made on disease transmission needs to be conducted. This is challenging and often beyond the technical capability of a country's ministry of health. External partners such as the WHO, research institutions, and universities have a key role to play in defining the evaluation testing to be conducted. They also provide funds and technical support for the evaluation work and, in some cases, laboratory testing facilities to conduct the large number of sample tests involved. In the LF elimination initiative, this work has been funded by a grant from the Bill & Melinda Gates Foundation. Evaluations are currently underway in many countries engaged in the LF elimination initiative to demonstrate that transmission has been interrupted, and that mass drug administration can be safety stopped.

Stopping an intervention is a critical decision. If terminated too early, it may be difficult to restart the program if necessary. Consequently, country program managers are (rightly) cautious about stopping treatment and tend to take a low-risk approach by continuing treatment. There is the risk that treatment could continue beyond the point where it is actually needed, with consequent wasted effort, resources, and drugs. The cost and effort required to conduct a thorough evaluation upon which to base the decision to stop treatment may, however, be more challenging than the decision to continue to treat. Thus, external support is needed to assist a program manager in establishing the scientific evidence that it is safe to stop.

Evaluation of Impact

Separate from monitoring the progress achieved by the program is the evaluation of the overall impact on public health and economies of the affected countries. Disease elimination and eradication initiatives make a significant impact on public health, both for the people treated and for those who are spared the disease because transmission has been interrupted. In addition to health benefits, there are also economic benefits which accrue to individuals and families and the wider national and world economies.

The LF elimination program, for example, has been implemented in over fifty countries for more than ten years. Ottesen et al. (2008) calculate that after the first eight years, the disease had been prevented in 6.6 million newborns who would have otherwise acquired LF. Furthermore, the program averted 1.4 million cases of hydrocele, 800,000 cases of lymphodema, and 4.4 million cases of subclinical disease. A follow-up paper by Chu et al. (2010) reported on the economic benefits of the LF elimination program. They estimate that USD 21.8 billion of direct economic benefits will be gained over the lifetime of the 31.4 million individuals who were treated during the first eight years of the program.

Such evaluations are challenging to perform. However, a robust analysis of health and economic benefits is a powerful advocacy tool to convince governments and donors of the value of investing in disease elimination and eradication programs. It also serves as a motivator to encourage current partners and donors to stay engaged in the program through to completion.

Budgeting and Cost Management

A key mechanism for the implementation of disease control, elimination, and eradication initiatives is budgeting and cost control. This is important both at the level of the international partnership and at the country level where the program is implemented.

At the international level, the partnership needs to budget for funds to perform their roles of supporting the country programs with technical guidance. It is also needed to provide the necessary tools such as purchased diagnostics, drugs, and vaccines.

At the country level, a program manager needs to develop a budget for the implementation activities and fund these using grants from external sources (if available) and government budget. In an ideal situation, the country ministry of health is able to establish a line in the health budget for the program which the program manager can access. However, experience shows that a budget line is not established by the government; thus the program is forced to live somewhat "hand to mouth," seeking approval of funds each year. This is inherently unpredictable, and many programs have suffered delays in conducting interventions due to late availability of funds. In worst cases, programs have simply not been able to progress, and treatments have been missed in certain years.

Data Management

A disease control, elimination, or eradication initiative generates an enormous amount of data on mapping, treatment interventions, and monitoring of impact. Effective data management is a vital mechanism but can be hugely complex. The required information originates at the peripheral level and must be captured and routed through to the national and international levels. Flows from peripheral agents through district and regional tiers of the health system to the national level are often beset with problems frequently associated with a lack of training, expertise, and suitable data management and transfer systems. Limited capacity in countries often means that most data is captured manually and physically transferred back to the program office. Thereafter, country program managers have to collate the data and provide reports to the ministry of health, donors, and WHO. These challenges are compounded at a WHO regional and global level, since the contributing countries often utilize different systems, resulting in huge challenges for coordination.

New activities are underway in several disease programs to employ modern information technology, such as mobile phones to speed up the capture and transfer of information. This is a new area that has yet to have a major impact on current disease initiatives.

Safety Monitoring and Reporting

Effective safety monitoring is an important mechanism that must be in place to support disease programs that utilize drugs or vaccines. Most drugs and vaccines have side effects, which are usually minor (e.g., headache or nausea); however, very occasionally severe adverse experiences (SAEs) can occur. An adverse event is defined by the U.S. Food and Drug Administration as any undesirable experience associated with the use of a medical product in a patient (U.S. FDA 2009). The event is classified as serious when patient outcome is fatal, life threatening, or disabling or involves the hospitalization of the patient.

Programs to control, eliminate, or eradicate diseases typically treat millions of people with drugs or vaccines. Thus it is vital to have an effective system to capture any reported SAEs. Reliable reporting helps raise confidence of populations in the drugs and vaccines that are used, and ensures that any reported incidents are taken seriously and investigated. Pharmaceutical companies are legally required to report all cases of SAEs so that the reports can be analyzed to detect any signals of potential safety issues. These reports must be made to the relevant regulatory authorities within a strict timetable.

WHO has published guidelines for SAE reporting in NTD programs, which include the forms to be completed for each reported incidence (WHO 2006d). These guidelines are useful for establishing and strengthening pharmaco-vigilance systems in countries where these mechanisms are weak. However, the

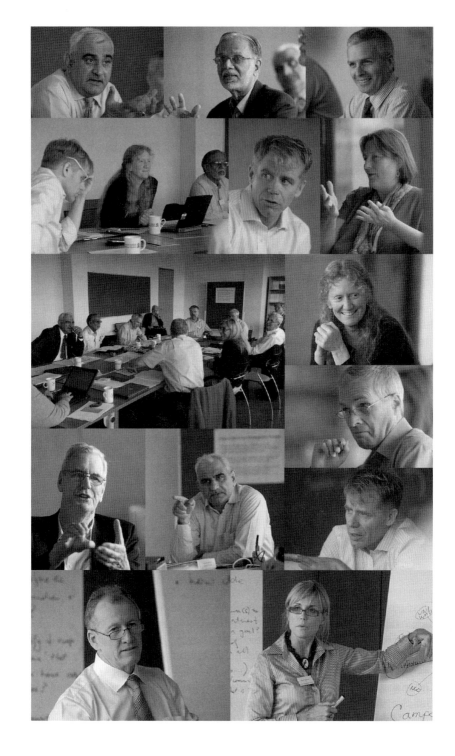

14

Group Report: Elements of Good Governance in Disease Eradication Initiatives

Kari Stoever, Chris Maher, R. Bruce Aylward,
Julie Jacobson, Ali Jaffer Mohamed,
T. Jacob John, Robert S. Scott, and Andy Wright

Abstract

This chapter identifies five key elements required to launch, execute, and manage a global eradication initiative, taking into consideration time, resources, and technical expertise in the context of the 21st century. The five elements include conducting a landscape analysis, obtaining the necessary commitments from a diverse group of stakeholders, constructing a framework to support the program, monitoring and managing the collaboration process, and incorporating research into the core operations of the program. Regardless of the type of organizational arrangement, there is a fundamental need to understand the changing dynamics of a program, both as a function of the evolution of the eradication program and the environment within which a global eradication effort operates. Recommendations in this chapter were informed by the lessons learned from the Global Polio Eradication Initiative, the Global Alliance to Eliminate Lymphatic Filariasis, and, to a lesser extent, the Guinea Worm Eradication Program and the groundwork being established around measles eradication.

Introduction

In the 21st century, before organizational arrangements are established, disease eradication programs will be subject to a series of prerequisite steps, such as meeting feasibility criteria and establishing a business case, to garner sufficient political will. A core group of stakeholders will need to champion the formative work and establish the initial mechanisms for collaboration. However, to broaden support and manage the collaboration process in a multicultural and nonhierarchical environment, a series of sequential steps are required to co-opt new constituents. Once sufficient buy-in has been achieved, structural arrangements should be identified to assist in facilitating work so that it can adapt to new data and embrace new technologies to achieve even more. The ultimate goal of any structural arrangement is to reduce bureaucracy and simplify work toward a common goal.

To identify, organize, and activate a diverse group of actors (agencies, stakeholders, individuals, and groups) in support of a global eradication effort, we subdivided the main question into two areas. The first addresses the precursors that would inform on the types of organizational arrangements to support a global, large-scale, and multiyear program. The second builds on these initial requirements and extrapolates from them the essential elements required to execute and manage a global eradication program.

We constructed a multidimensional framework that can be applied to any disease eradication or elimination initiative. Components of the framework include functional areas and governance issues that address accountability, leadership, monitoring, and risk management. The framework focuses on the global organizational arrangements but is scalable and can be applied toward regional programs or smaller-scale global eradication efforts for diseases such as yaws.

The Critical Role of Scanning the Environment and Conducting a Stakeholder Analysis

Once the technical feasibility and investment case has been established to eradicate a disease, a thorough scan of the environment needs to be conducted. The scan enables decision makers to understand the external environment and the interconnections of its various sectors as well as to translate this understanding into the planning and decision-making processes (Fahey et al. 1981). Basic components of the analysis include:

- assessment of political will at the global, regional, and national levels,
- financing trends in global health,
- general economic trends,
- assessment of perceptions and demand for eradication programs, and
- a list of actors required to launch and support the program.

Once the key components of the analysis have been completed, the data needs to be analyzed and presented in a SWOT analysis[1] framework; critical gaps should be identified, and a decision made to move to the initial strategic planning phase. The strategic plan will focus on the launch phase of the eradication

---

[1] SWOT analysis is a strategic planning method used to evaluate the strengths, weaknesses, opportunities, and threats involved in a project.

program and on obtaining the necessary commitments from key stakeholders in support of a resolution.

The identification of key actors is a critical step in understanding how you create buy-in and from whom it must be obtained to align the various actors within the organizational framework. Each actor in the system is grouped into core functional areas:

- national governments,
- interested parties (e.g., national governments, UN agencies, technical agencies, civil society groups, affected communities, NGOs),
- a group of core partners or agencies who share leadership and responsibilities toward achieving the goal ("spearheading" partners),
- influencers (e.g., media, champions, academia, think tanks, advocates),
- industry,
- enablers (e.g., funders, policy makers, implementing organizations, technical agencies), and
- disablers.

Understanding the role of each actor in the broader environment allows the program to start thinking through the various ways key actors will be engaged, consent, and interact throughout the course of the eradication program. It is important to recognize the changing dynamics of the program throughout its life cycle. Structures will need to be built as well as eliminated over time to meet the changing needs of the program, so as to keep the partnership lean and efficient, recognizing as well that the roles of partners may shift over time.

Obtaining the Necessary Commitments to Eradicate a Disease in the 21st Century

Engaging stakeholders in the formative stages of a disease eradication program to obtain their buy-in and support means that the old way of initiating a global eradication effort (i.e., through the mechanism of the World Health Assembly) may require reengineering. While we determined that the World Health Assembly resolution is essential to any global eradication effort, we also agreed that it was not sufficient to achieve the requisite buy-in from a diverse group of stakeholders—the core group that will ultimately be responsible for launching and managing the program as well as maintaining momentum to achieve eradication. For future initiatives, multiple mechanisms may be needed to obtain commitment, ranging from formal legal arrangements and informed consent to memorandums of understanding and other nonlegally binding commitments.

Prior to obtaining a formal global resolution, spearheading partners should have completed an environmental scan, a feasibility analysis, an investment case, and an outreach strategy to engage various actors and stakeholders and obtain the necessary commitment to launch the initiative. Two aspects of an effective engagement strategy are: (a) understanding the overlap of vital interests and (b) creating a shared sense of local impact.

The earlier stakeholders are engaged and the more actively they participate in the decision, the more likely they are to withstand the inevitable trials and challenges associated with a long-term eradication effort. Ignoring the vital interests and spheres of influence that actors and stakeholders have in committing to the goal can undermine and derail the partnership, adding years onto the program and potentially billions of dollars to the overall costs.

Constructing a Multidimensional Framework to Support an Eradication Program

To operate effectively, an explicit formative stage is needed for each eradication initiative. Galvanizing commitment around the goal, applying resources, and establishing organizing principles provides a more resilient, adaptable type of order than is found in a conventional hierarchical arrangement or public-private partnership (Kelly et al. 2007). These initial efforts will lead to the identification of spearheading partners.

Spearheading partners have several key functions that establish the foundation of the framework as well as the ways in which actors and key stakeholders interact to coordinate activities within the broader partnership (Figure 14.1). Because of its critical role as the primary interface with national governments, particularly in coordination and support of countries for implementation (Figure 14.2), the WHO is well positioned to be an essential spearheading partner. It often acts as a convener and consensus builder; it provides technical support to countries and partners and will ultimately certify eradication.

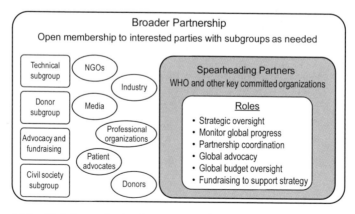

Figure 14.1   Global organizational arrangement in support of country-led eradication efforts.

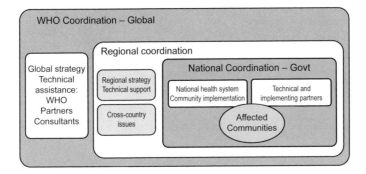

Figure 14.2   Technical and implementation support structure of national eradication programs.

However, the WHO does not necessarily have to serve as the sole lead agency in an eradication effort. Often, an inspirational champion emerges to galvanize momentum and inspire collective motivation among partners. Based on lessons learned in the polio program, various spearheading partners may lead at different points in time. Flexibility and the need for shared leadership is a key determinant of success in sustaining an eradication program.

To lead successfully, spearheading partners must ensure that key leadership attributes are present in one or more of the organizations. These include the role of the Good Samaritan or neutral broker (e.g., Rotary in polio), the coordinator, the champion, the technical expert, and a strong figurehead to represent the partnership and maintain momentum. Any spearheading partner may fulfill one or more of these attributes. These roles become the "glue" in the eradication initiative and provide the leadership and stability required to manage challenges and survive a crisis.

Monitoring and Managing the Architecture of the Eradication Program

Once the spearheading partners have been identified and the formative stage of the partnership completed, the partnership must identify and implement processes to execute and manage the eradication program successfully. The spearheading organizations are responsible for managing the progress of the program and reporting to their constituencies on a regular basis. Spearheading partners organize and manage at the global level, and their key responsibilities include:

- strategic planning,
- advocacy and fundraising,
- ensuring the research agenda is developed and managed,

- coordinating the partnership,
- program monitoring,
- risk management, and
- funding flow and resource allocation (based on the strategic plan).

Technical, research, and funding agencies converge around the global strategic plan to prioritize activities and support with resources. A clear process for managing resources needs to be determined in the formative stages of the partnership. Where multiple funding avenues exist, a group of spearheading representatives provides direction to the various funders in support of the strategic plan. Activities assigned to the spearheading partners can be delegated to one or more partners outside of the spearheading group. Drawing on experience from the polio program, we recommend that the management structure of the spearheading partners meet electronically on a regular basis (e.g., every 14 days) and in person at least twice a year, on a rotational basis at each stakeholder's head office. The broader stakeholder group should convene once a year. In addition, a strong management component needs to be built into these programs from the very beginning, with regular and timely monitoring and reporting back to the constituents.

The spearheading partners receive requests for funding and allocate resources based on feedback from regional- and national-level coordinating bodies. These bodies are responsible for establishing annual plans and budgets; in addition, they provide the spearheading partners with critical data that will identify threats to achieving eradication. The regional- and national-level coordinating bodies work with local stakeholders (e.g., national ministries, donors, nongovernmental organizations, civil society, industry) in support of national plans, and play a pivotal role in organizing the work and aligning stakeholder activities nationally. The coordinating groups also play a role in maintaining political will with national ministries as well as monitoring progress and identifying problems.

Accountability within the program depends largely on the ability to monitor and manage in a complex and constantly changing environment. Thus, an independent monitoring process—one that reports back to the leaders of the spearheading organizations—is essential. This independent monitoring group provides an objective assessment of the program and thus technical expertise needs to be embedded within the group. The group would advise the senior leaders of the spearheading organizations on risk, management approaches, and strategies to improve the performance of the program annually.

Research as a Core Component of an Eradication Program

The central and important role of research has been clearly demonstrated in historical attempts to eliminate or eradicate disease. Research should focus on the key areas where a program can fail. It should build on a strong monitoring and evaluation component that is always looking with a critical mind toward innovative problem solving. The research agenda becomes one of the core functions managed by the spearheading group, with technical and academic groups playing a pivotal role in implementing the research agenda.

To ensure that an eradication program is equipped to monitor, manage, and mitigate threats to the program, a framework for establishing research priorities needs to be included at the onset of an eradication program and included in the strategic plan and budget (Figure 14.3). Early considerations must be given to define what success would look like and how it would be measured. Looking at the areas of potential failure within the framework, research provides a valuable tool for managing risk throughout the life of the program. Particular attention should be given to how new data, tools, and technologies will be integrated into the program in a timely fashion. The research agenda should be proactive and responsive to innovations from the field and other disciplines, and needs to be capable of learning from a strong monitoring, evaluation, and reporting system.

Final Thoughts on Designing the Operational Structures of a Global Eradication Program

The 21st century offers unprecedented opportunity to solve some of the world's greatest challenges, including the eradication of diseases that affect humans. Disease eradication is more feasible now than ever before, with improved interventions, diagnostics, technology, and advances in social science and management theory. What is ultimately required to leverage this opportunity are new perspectives, novel ways of collaborating, and innovative ways of engaging a broader set of actors in designing and implementing those solutions.

Social media, cause marketing, tax incentives, financial engineering, and many other mechanisms exist to complement traditional donor government

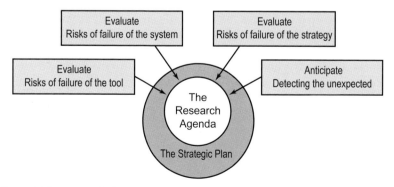

Figure 14.3   Research framework and placement within strategic plan.

and multinational agency financial support. We expect that globalization and technology will increasingly drive new fundraising mechanisms to boost resources for global health programs. Driven by individuals who make small contributions to charities or causes, microphilanthropy has the potential of integrating into online and offline technology platforms to become a part of the donor culture. Disciplines such as marketing, branding, advertising, and public relations will continue to drive awareness and engage individuals in global health issues. New civil society groups will emerge in virtual communities. Over time, these communities will improve their effectiveness in mobilizing collective action around a cause.

Social media tools, such as Facebook, Twitter, LinkedIn, YouTube and MySpace, have changed the way we view our world and the communities in which we interact and engage. It is now commonplace for strangers to align along a common mission in 140 characters or less (Twitter) or to "become a fan" of a cause or point of view (Facebook) or to take the initiative and, through video, document real-time events as they unfold and inform the world (YouTube). At the individual level, we are all now equipped with a variety of one-to-the-masses communication tools. The explosion in social media, coupled with a growing awareness that communities need to be united in creating solutions to the problems that plague our planet, provide new opportunities for an eradication program to collaborate with civil society. Technology offers the possibility of taking an issue to communities broadly and quickly, to achieve consensus and engagement, and to find creative solutions to problems.

We believe that fundamental to the success of future eradication programs will be new ways of thinking about the importance of people to the process of eradication, and not just the availability of tools to eradicate disease. New online communities will strengthen the ability to collaborate and share best practices, and access to information will empower actors across the broader community to form opinions, react to challenges, and support the generation of new ideas (see Stoever, this volume). Equally, however, the easy access to information can lead to the quick spread of rumors and misinformation, which can ultimately slow or hinder progress. Thus, eradication programs must be aware and prepared to address the new challenges as well as the advantages inherent in our modern technological age.

We hope that in any future eradication initiative, new training and management tools powered by information will help people to build skills and competencies, and that empowered by a more decentralized decision-making structure, individual responsibility will increase as more responsibility is placed on individuals at all levels within communities and organizations.

We have entered an age of new possibilities. To move eradication efforts into the 21st century, we must embrace a new concept of partnership—one that is nimble and flexible based on shared leadership. This partnership must harness the new tools available in social and technical sectors, and constantly challenge our assumptions and adapt to allow programs to evolve. If we are successful in this, we may hopefully enter the 22nd century having prevailed over additional diseases that plague humankind.

Recommendations

1. Eradication efforts in the 21st century must be based on a partnership of agencies and actors. They must incorporate the key elements needed for success in a flexible and dynamic structure, so that each partner is able to contribute to the shared success. At the core of this partnership should be a spearheading group of agencies, committed to achieving the eradication goal.
2. Strong business management and leadership skills are required to support eradication programs and should be established in the spearheading partner organizations during the formative stages of a disease eradication initiative.
3. To ensure global accountability, the World Health Assembly should provide a forum for an annual report to stakeholders on progress achieved toward eradication.
4. Research should be embraced as part of the strategic plan for eradication and should be actively used to update and modify the program for success.
5. Spearheading partners should communicate and convene frequently to facilitate collaboration and to negotiate changing roles and responsibilities.
6. The strengthening of health systems is an important objective for any eradication effort, but efforts to strengthen health systems should be within the context of the eradication program; the onus is on the broader health sector to take advantage of opportunities any eradication effort provides to strengthen health systems.
7. A strong central advisory body consisting of highly qualified and experienced people should provide technical guidance for global eradication efforts.
8. An independent body of respected and competent people should be formed as an independent monitoring group to assess progress toward the eradication goal for all stakeholders including the spearheading partners; their assessments should form the basis of reports to the World Health Assembly.

Disease Eradication
and Health Systems

15

Integration of Eradication Initiatives and Health Systems

Alan R. Hinman

Abstract

A wide range of strategies can be used to deliver health interventions, from single interventions to comprehensive preventive and curative services. Increasingly, policy makers, donors, and other development agencies are advocating the integration of interventions to achieve a comprehensive health system. This chapter considers the relative merits and contributions of single interventions and health systems, the opportunities and challenges for categorical programs in a health sector reform environment, the evidence on interactions between elimination/eradication initiatives and health systems, and the global movement toward integration.

The introduction of new vaccines has had many positive impacts on both immunization and health systems. These impacts, however, have not automatically been positive or negative. Characteristics of successful integration of child and maternal health services with immunization programs are (a) program compatibility (i.e., appropriate matching of programs based on staff skill requirements, program objectives, recommended timing of interventions, target populations, and drug/treatment characteristics), (b) existence of a robust immunization service, (c) support from key stakeholders, and (d) decentralization of health services.

At present, approximately 100 global health initiatives address a range of problems, from HIV/AIDS, trachoma, and meningitis, to reproductive health, health policy, and systems. Several of these initiatives feature periodic mass distribution of drugs or vaccines, often reaching people who would otherwise not be served by existing ongoing services. Still, these initiatives may divert health personnel from other duties.

Integrating comprehensive and categorical programs brings advantages as well as challenges. Careful planning is needed to ensure that targeted approaches and the development objectives for health systems are met in ways that maximize positive synergies while minimizing potential conflicts. Specific approaches and indicators are needed to help us achieve the common goal of preventing illness and saving lives.

Introduction

Many interventions (e.g., immunizations, prenatal care, tuberculosis treatment, sexually transmitted disease treatment, and family planning services) have been shown to be effective as well as cost-effective in preventing disease, disability, and death. However, they are not uniformly applied throughout the world; poor countries typically have the lowest rate of implementation due to a lack of human or financial resources and system capacity. As a result, in 2010, approximately 7.7 million children under the age of 5 years died (Rajaratnam et al. 2010). Of the estimated 10 million child deaths in 2000, analysis indicated that 63% of these deaths could have been avoided if proven and cost-effective interventions, which were demonstrated to be feasible to implement in developing countries, had been applied (Black et al. 2003; Jones et al. 2003).

Health interventions can be delivered along a spectrum of strategies:

- single intervention (e.g., smallpox vaccination, malaria treatment),
- integration of similar interventions (e.g., Expanded Program on Immunization, or EPI),
- opportunistic (or "convenience") integration with interventions that have different goals, but which can be delivered in the same manner (e.g., adding distribution of insecticide-treated bed nets to existing delivery systems for immunization),
- integration of a package of services which may or may not have the same delivery strategy and similar aims (e.g., Integrated Management of Childhood Illnesses, IMCI), and
- full integration of all clinical preventive and curative services (e.g., comprehensive primary care).

Over the past century, programs have been developed at national, regional, and global levels to address individual health problems or interventions (e.g., immunization). The most successful global intervention to date has been the global eradication of smallpox. Since 1974, the EPI, which is coordinated by the World Health Organization (WHO), has provided a basic set of immunizations (BCG, DTP, OPV, and measles) to infants around the world (WHO 2010b). More recently, hepatitis B and *Haemophilus influenzae* type b vaccines have been added, and rotavirus and pneumococcal conjugate vaccines will soon be introduced.

Increasingly, policy makers, donors, and other development agencies have advocated integrating selected interventions or broader integration to achieve a comprehensive health system. WHO describes health systems as containing six building blocks (WHO 2007a): service delivery; health workforce; information; medical products, vaccines, and technologies; financing; and leadership and governance (stewardship).

In this chapter, I discuss the relative merits and contributions of single interventions and health systems, the opportunities and challenges for and Development (ACSD) program in three countries in West Africa: Benin, Ghana, and Mali. The ACSD program provided packages of interventions:

- Immunization plus (EPI+) adds vitamin A supplementation and distribution of insecticide-treated bed nets.
- Antenatal care (ANC+) provides intermittent preventive treatment of malaria in pregnant women, tetanus immunization during pregnancy, and supplementation with iron and folic acid during pregnancy and vitamin A postpartum.
- Improved management of pneumonia, malaria, and diarrhea (IMCI+) promotes exclusive breastfeeding up to 6 months, improved and integrated management of children with pneumonia, malaria, and diarrhea, and household consumption of iodized salt.

Although there were decreases in mortality in children <5 years in the ACSD areas, the decreases were not greater than those in comparison areas. Bryce et al. (2010:572) concluded:

> The ACSD project did not accelerate child survival in Benin and Mali focus districts relative to comparison areas, probably because coverage for effective treatment interventions for malaria and pneumonia were not accelerated, causes of neonatal deaths and under nutrition were not addressed, and stock shortages of insecticide-treated nets restricted the potential effect of this intervention.

In a study of the interactions between a multi-intervention neglected tropical diseases initiative in Mali (four drugs targeting five diseases) and the country health system at the health center level, Cavalli et al. (2010:2) found at the local level that

> campaign effects of care delivery differed across health services. In robust and well staffed health centres, the personnel successfully facilitated mass drug distribution while running routine consultations, an overall service functioning benefitted from programme resources. In more fragile health centres however, additional program workload severely disturbed access to regular care, and [they] observed operational problems affecting the quality of mass drug distribution. Strong health services appeared to be profitable to the NTD control program as well as to general care.

They concluded that "health system strengthening will not result from the sum of selective global interventions but requires a comprehensive approach."

Global Movement toward Integration

Over the past 20–25 years, several global initiatives have been launched that have attracted large-scale funding from development agencies, multilateral institutions, and foundations. For example, the Polio Eradication Initiative (Polio Eradication Initiative 2010a), which is nearing achievement of its target, has expended more than USD 6 billion over the period 1985–2010. The Onchocerciasis Control Initiative, which features donations of Mectizan® (ivermectin) from Merck, has provided more than 700 million treatments since 1987 (Mectizan Donation Program 2010). Innovative mechanisms were developed to fund these initiatives, including the Global Fund to fight AIDS, Tuberculosis, and Malaria (GFATM), which has provided USD 19.3 billion since 2002 for more than 572 programs in 144 countries. GFATM provides a quarter of all international financing for global activities against HIV/AIDS, two-thirds for tuberculosis, and three-quarters for malaria (GFATM 2010). As of August 2008, the GAVI Alliance had approved a total of USD 3.7 billion to countries for the period 2000–2015 to support introduction and use of new and underused vaccines as well as to support immunization and health system strengthening in the poorest countries of the world (GAVI Alliance 2010a). Several of these initiatives feature periodic mass distribution of drugs, vaccines, or other modalities, which are often successful in reaching people who do not normally have access to existing health services. At the same time, however, the campaigns may divert health personnel from other duties to participate in the campaign.

At present, there are approximately 100 global health initiatives (GHIs) which address a variety of health issues, ranging from HIV/AIDS, trachoma, and meningitis to reproductive health, health policy, and systems. GHIs represent "a concerted effort by several countries to finance the delivery of specific types of services for priority health problems that arise in many low-income countries" (WHO Maximizing Positive Synergies Collaborative Group 2009:2140). They bring significant levels of funding to target specific health issues. This can have a significant positive effect on the condition being targeted, but it can also distort a country's ability to set priorities and allocate staff in a planned, rational manner.

Reviewing the patterns of financing for global health activities from 1990–2007, Ravishankar et al. (2009) found a major increase, from USD 5.6 billion to USD 21.8 billion, in overall development assistance during this time. Although GHIs constituted a major part, funding for broader health system development also increased. As development assistance increased, so did the call to make assistance more effective. The 2005 Paris Declaration on Aid Effectiveness set out a series of mutual commitments by donors and partner countries (OECD 2008a) in the following areas:

- Ownership: partner countries exercise effective leadership over their development policies and strategies and coordinate development actions.
- Alignment: donors base their overall support on partner countries' national development strategies, institutions, and procedures.
- Harmonization: donors' actions are more harmonized, transparent, and collectively effective.

- Managing for results: aid is managed and implemented in a way that focuses on the desired results, and information is used to improve decision making.
- Mutual accountability: donors and partners are accountable for development results.

Problems may result, however, from the large-scale influx of additional resources to a country brought about by GHIs. These resources can be huge relative to national budgets. They may exceed the absorptive capacity of the country's health system and create distortions in the allocation of the health workforce (Tangcharoensathien and Patcharanarumol 2010). In addition, GHIs may not adequately address the existing bottlenecks in a country's health system.

Given the unacceptably high, continuing burden of preventable child deaths, interest has increased in broadening the scope of health initiatives to deliver concurrently a number of interventions, primarily through what was described above as opportunistic integration. For example, in 2008, measles supplemental activities in 17 African countries also included vitamin A in 16 countries (>57 million doses), deworming in 10 countries (23.9 million doses), insecticide-treated bed nets (ITNs) in 6 countries (3.4 million nets), and oral polio vaccine (OPV) in 9 countries.

The WHO Maximizing Positive Synergies Collaborative Group (2009) has developed a conceptual framework of the interaction between GHIs and country health systems (Figure 15.1). They found that the evidence for the effect of GHIs and access and uptake of other health services that are not the specific target of their investments is weak and inconclusive, representing primarily associations rather than cause-and-effect relationships. Positive potential interactions could be that GHI services revitalize health facilities, increase reliability of supplies and availability of qualified personnel, and encourage community demand. In addition, GHIs might be able to free up resources so

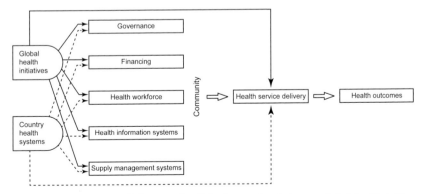

Figure 15.1   Conceptual framework of the interaction between global health initiatives and country health systems (WHO Maximizing Positive Synergies Collaborative Group 2009; reprinted from *The Lancet* with permission from Elsevier).

that other problems can be addressed. Potentially negative interactions include disruption of basic health services as a result of needing to use existing staff for campaigns, insistence on stand-alone information systems that may not be compatible with country health information systems, and use of duplicate supply chains.

The WHO Maximizing Positive Synergies Collaborative Group came to two conclusions. First, GHIs and country health systems are not independent; they are inextricably linked. Second, their interactions are so complex that generalizations may be dangerous. On this basis, the group developed the following recommendations:

1. Infuse the health systems-strengthening agenda with the sense of ambition and speed that has characterized GHIs.
2. Extend the targets of GHIs and agree on indicators for health systems strengthening.
3. Improve alignment of planning processes and resource allocations among GHIs, as well as between GHIs and country health systems.
4. Generate more reliable data for the costs and benefits of strengthening health systems and evidence to inform additional and complementary investments to those of GHIs.
5. Ensure a rise in national and global health financing, and in more predictable financing to support the sustainable and equitable growth of health systems.

In further discussion on maximizing positive synergies between health systems and GHIs, participants from a conference in Venice issued a statement, now known as the Venice statement. It acknowledges "that the impact of global health initiatives on health outcomes and health systems, though variable, has been positive on balance and has helped to draw attention to deficiencies in health systems" (Horton 2009:11) and concludes with two calls to action:

> Call on the World Health Organization, drawing on its standards setting and convening roles, to work with partners to enhance alignment and further coordinate technical support to countries for implementation of country-driven and context-specific health systems-strengthening policies and plans.

> Call on all national governments and development partners to mobilize required additional resources through existing and innovative means to accelerate and sustain health systems strengthening, inclusive of disease-specific work, to reach the shared goal of saving lives and improving the health of all people.

In a thoughtful review of the issues that surround the vertical and horizontal delivery of services, Oliveira-Cruz et al. (2003:83) concluded:

> Vertical and horizontal approaches do not have to be seen as mutually exclusive but rather as complementary strategies, thus pointing to the need to discard the dichotomy of one versus the other. Expanding access to priority health

services requires the concerted use of both vertical and horizontal approaches, in accordance with the capacity of health systems as it changes over time.

One of the four aims of the Global Immunization Vision and Strategy, developed by WHO and UNICEF in 2005, is "to integrate other critical health interventions with immunization" (GIVS 2011).

The International Health Partnership and related initiatives seek "to achieve better health results by mobilizing donor countries and other development partners around a single country-led national health strategy" (IHP+ 2010). Guided by the principles of the Paris Declaration on Aid Effectiveness and the Accra Agenda for Action, IHP+ was launched in September 2007 to better harmonize donor funding commitments and improve the way international agencies, donors, and developing countries work together to develop and implement national health plans.

The GAVI Alliance recently updated its strategic goals. One of them is to "contribute to strengthening the capacity of integrated health systems to deliver immunization" (GAVI Alliance 2010b).

Despite the continuing debate about health systems and GHIs and the growing movement toward harmonization or integration of programs, there continues to be great interest in GHIs. For example, at the 63rd World Health Assembly in May 2010, member States endorsed a series of interim targets set for 2015 as milestones toward the eventual global eradication of measles. Success in achieving the measles 2015 targets is a key issue, if the Millennium Development Goal 4 (to reduce child mortality) is to be reached. In her opening address to the 63rd World Health Assembly, Margaret Chan, Director-General of the WHO, said (Chan 2010):

> We need horizontal and we need vertical approaches. We need to scale up the delivery of commodities, and we need to strengthen the fundamental capacities that allow us to do so. We need coherence in policies, within and beyond the health sector, and we need complementarity of efforts....International donors, partners, and governments themselves have failed to rally around national health policies, strategies, and priorities. This contributes to fragmentation, duplication, added demands and costs, and defeats national ownership. We have learned this. How can we scale up interventions or aim for universal coverage when health systems in so many countries are on the verge of collapse? Or when the world faces a shortage of 4 million doctors, nurses, and other health personnel? Weak health systems blunt the power of global health initiatives to reach their goals. Weak health systems are wasteful. They waste money, and dilute the return on investments. They waste money when regulatory systems fail to control the price and quality of medicines or the costs of care in the private sector. They waste training when workers are lured away by better working conditions or better pay. They waste efficiency when needless procedures are performed, or when essential procedures are precluded by interruptions in the supply chain. They waste opportunities for poverty reduction when poor people are driven even deeper into poverty by the costs of care or the failure of preventive services. Above all, weak health systems waste lives. This problem is now recognized

by countries and donors alike, and it is being addressed by a range of new and existing initiatives, including several global health initiatives. Though designed to deliver specific health outcomes, these initiatives now recognize that meeting their goals depends on a well-functioning health system. In my view, this shift of attention is nothing short of revolutionary.

In a presentation at the Harvard School of Public Health on July 16, 2008, Carissa Etienne reported that 11% of GAVI support and 35% of Global Fund support had gone for health systems strengthening. Other indications of the effort to integrate GHI with other activities include the explicit effort to strengthen general immunization services as laid out in the Strategic Plan 2010–2012 of the Polio Eradication Initiative (2010b:42, 44):

> A 2001 survey of over 1,000 GPEI staff documented that 100% of national staff and >90% of international staff were already engaged in routine immunization and surveillance for other diseases of public health importance. These staff devoted, on average, 22% and 44% of their time, respectively, to such activities. With >95% of WHO's immunization staff in GAVI-eligible countries funded by the GPEI, this infrastructure has been critical to the rapid scale-up of the work of the GAVI Alliance in sub-Saharan Africa and Asia, especially for the introduction of new and under-used vaccines....It is expected that GPEI staff will on average spend a minimum of 25% of their time on systems strengthening.

Another indication of the move toward integration was provided by the United States, in an announcement by President Obama in May 2009 (Kates 2010). This global health initiative will commit USD 63 billion over six years (2009–2014), with USD 51 billion allocated for HIV, TB, and malaria and USD12 billion designated for other global health priorities, including maternal health, child health, nutrition, family planning/reproductive health, neglected tropical diseases, and health systems strengthening. The four main implementation components of this initiative are:

1. Do more of what works, promote proven approaches.
2. Build on and expand existing platforms.
3. Innovate for results.
4. Collaborate for impact/promote country ownership.

Conclusion

No matter how one views the integration of health systems and eradication/elimination initiatives, integration is happening. Many papers have been written about the relative merits of targeted vs. integrated approaches. Most recognize that there are potentially both advantages and challenges in integrating comprehensive and categorical programs. Many agree that the challenge is to plan carefully so that targeted approaches and health systems development objectives are met in ways that maximize the positive synergies and minimize potential conflicts. What we now need is to agree on specific approaches and indicators (e.g., along the lines of those of Wallace et al. 2009) and use those to help us achieve our common goals of preventing illness and saving lives.

Acknowledgment

The author is indebted to Uche Amazigo for suggestions in conceptualizing this paper and to Aaron Wallace for important information on his studies of integration of interventions.

16

How Can Elimination and Eradication Initiatives Best Contribute to Health Systems Strengthening?

Stewart Tyson and Robin Biellik

Abstract

This chapter reviews major developments in global health over recent decades, in particular, the influence of targeted disease elimination or eradication initiatives on efforts to build sustainable health services in developing countries. It is based on a review of published literature, comments of health care workers, and personal opinion.

The health and development landscape has become increasingly complex with many more actors, far greater funding levels and many, often competing, demands on limited country capacity. As greater attention and resources have focused on specific diseases and interventions, long-standing tensions between targeted and comprehensive approaches to improve health have been exacerbated. Despite positive interactions, much more could be achieved to strengthen health systems.

At the outset, future disease elimination/eradication initiatives should consider potential impacts on the key components of the health system and actively pursue efforts to minimize negative effects and maximize benefits during implementation.

Introduction

Efforts to eliminate/eradicate communicable diseases have been pursued for more than a century. In the 1950s and 1960s, breakthroughs in pharmaceuticals and vector control were translated into malaria, smallpox, and other disease control initiatives (Mills 1983). These occurred at a time of faith in the potential of targeted delivery of solutions based on good science to realize ambitious global goals as well as what were perceived to be quick wins in global health.

Programs were introduced into basic health care systems where immunization was typically limited to BCG and smallpox, where there was no effective national disease surveillance, and where population coverage with essential health care services was limited. Despite the early failure of efforts to eradicate yaws and malaria, the success of smallpox eradication in 1977, after a decade of intense effort, led the World Health Assembly (WHA) to pass resolutions for the eradication of guinea worm in 1986 and polio in 1988. Today, disease elimination initiatives are also underway in large parts of the world against lymphatic filariasis, onchocerciasis, malaria, and measles. In 2008, the WHA tasked the World Health Organization (WHO) to report on prospects for measles eradication. The polio and guinea worm eradication programs have been ongoing for more than twenty years and, in spite of recent reversals, there remains optimism that eradication can be achieved. The literature indicates that these programs have had both positive and negative impacts on national health systems.

Eradication/elimination initiatives share many characteristics with the increasing number of targeted disease-specific control programs that have been launched over the past decade and with which they interact. Here we review the impact of such programs on health systems and suggest ways in which any negative impact can be minimized and benefits maximized.

Overview of Influences on Country Health Systems

International institutions have long influenced global health policy and the development of health services in developing countries. In 1978, the Alma-Ata International Conference on Primary Health Care promoted comprehensive primary health care (WHO 1978). As initially articulated, this revolutionized the way health was interpreted and radically changed models for organizing and delivering care. It aimed to influence the determinants of health that arise in nonhealth sectors and influenced the shift of public health from a narrow biomedical slant to a view of health today which recognizes the central importance of social, economic, and political determinants.

Only two years after Alma-Ata, Walsh and Warren (1980) proposed selective primary health care as an interim strategy for disease control in developing countries. This implicitly considered comprehensive primary health care as too ambitious and focused instead on the provision of a limited number of programs selected on the grounds of cost-effectiveness. This led to the promotion of an array of selective programs in countries which often had limited capacity to deliver. Since then, the tensions between comprehensive (or horizontal) and selective (or targeted/vertical) approaches to improve health outcomes have continued to influence the global health agenda.

Disease elimination/eradication initiatives are time limited and organized in circumscribed programs. Mass campaigns can effectively address diseases that are widespread, have a high prevalence and incidence, and affect a high proportion of the population. With a well-defined scope, clear objectives, and relatively short duration, such initiatives can deliver quick results. Mass campaigns are straightforward to manage and monitor and are able to attract substantial donor support. Because they have often operated through delivery channels parallel to existing systems, critics in many developing countries have perceived them as diverting human and financial resources from resource-constrained systems, to the detriment of the overall health systems development. Time-limited elimination/eradication initiatives in an underfunded sector can create islands of excellence that place substantial pressures on the health delivery system. In contrast, the health delivery system is a permanent fixture; in theory (but rarely in practice) it is comprehensive, able to adjust to shifting disease patterns, and embedded in community life. The integration of targeted initiatives into the mainstream health system can, in principle, result in greater efficiency, place the initiative within the context of other competing priorities, and generate more sustainable political and community support. The evidence below suggests that these potential gains, however, remain to be realized.

Early elimination/eradication initiatives were implemented in an environment where the aid architecture was far simpler; fewer players were involved at both the international and country level. Developing countries accommodated a number of targeted programs alongside ongoing efforts to develop broad-based health services. Health is just one of many development priorities. With few exceptions, domestic health budgets have increased modestly or fallen behind minimal levels, as defined by the WHO. Economic crises, debt repayment, conflict, and poor governance have exacerbated poverty and inequality and weakened health systems in most developing countries. Policies such as structural adjustment, designed to improve economic stability, often led to cuts in public spending. The globalization of labor markets in the 1990s increased the migration of skilled health workers, and the HIV/AIDS pandemic further undermined already weakened health systems (Rockefeller Foundation 2003; WHO 2006b).

Since the mid-1990s, concerns have been raised over the ineffectiveness of much aid. Proposals have been made for new approaches that provide direct financial support to governments to implement their own prioritized national development plans (Cassels 1997; OECD 2005; IHP+ 2007; DFID 2007).

The Millennium Declaration in 2000 influenced the establishment or expansion of a number of high-profile global health initiatives. This led to massive increases in resources which targeted a limited number of diseases or interventions, particularly against HIV/AIDS, tuberculosis, malaria, and childhood immunization. The expansion of such initiatives in recent years dramatically altered the landscape of aid and public health. Most global health initiatives pursue disease- or intervention-specific agendas in an environment where country health systems struggle to achieve universal coverage with basic services. This is particularly the case in sub-Saharan Africa and South

Asia, where global investments in health have been largely driven by single-disease advocates and commodities.

Although new resources, partners, technical capacity, and political commitment were welcomed, some critics argued that increased efforts to meet disease-specific targets exacerbated the burden on fragile health systems. In 2003, Oxfam published a warning to the Global Fund to Fight AIDS, Tuberculosis and Malaria (GFATM), advising them to put in place programs designed to strengthen existing health systems, to ensure effectiveness and sustainable impact. The overconcentration of resources for specific programs left other areas underresourced and, where they existed, undermined sector-wide approaches (Oxfam 2002).

Pearson and colleagues highlighted that much disease-specific funding in Cambodia was neither aligned to the national health priorities nor to the national burden of disease. While the national plan prioritized primary health care and provision of a minimum health service package, most (60%) donor funding was allocated to HIV/AIDS and other infectious diseases (Pearson et al. 2008). In 2004, a high-level forum evaluated efforts to achieve the Millennium Development Goals for health and identified shortfalls in the health workforce, lack of donor coordination, and weak information systems as critical barriers to progress (WHO 2004).

The Global Alliance on Vaccines and Immunization (GAVI) recognized early that new generations of vaccines could not be introduced into weak or nonfunctional immunization systems, which had deteriorated since the end of the global push for universal childhood immunization in the 1980s. Thus GAVI introduced a flexible performance-related payment linked to improvements in immunization coverage. The financing mechanisms of the two largest initiatives, GAVI and GFATM, evolved to provide specific financing windows to strengthen health systems. Critics argued that these systems-strengthening funds were selective in targeting the system functions essential for implementation of the global health initiative programs and that they emphasized short-term rather than long-term contributions to systems strengthening.

In recent years, countries and donors have increasingly recognized the need to invest in building sustainable health systems to address all the major causes of ill health and disease, including other communicable diseases, neglected issues that contribute substantially to the burden of disease (e.g., reproductive health including maternal health), neglected tropical diseases (NTDs) such as filiarisais and onchocerciasis, mental health, and the rapidly mounting burden of noncommunicable diseases. The Millennium Development Goals for health will not be achieved without a more concerted and streamlined approach to improving health (IHP+ 2009).

It is possible that ever-evolving donor strategies to improve global health over the past thirty years have inadvertently contributed to the dysfunction of some health systems, which in the poorest of countries fail to deliver the most basic health care. Thus, on the thirtieth anniversary of Alma-Ata, the WHO has called for a return to the principles of primary health care (WHO 2008c).

The Effectiveness of Aid

The increased profile and resources for global health have coincided with mounting concern over the ineffectiveness of much aid. In comparison with other sectors, donor assistance for health tends to be highly volatile, fluctuating from one year to another, and is poorly coordinated between donors. The large number of health initiatives and competing implementing agencies results in high transaction costs for government. Ministries of Health commonly complain of distortion, duplication, poor coordination, and inadequate sequencing of activities (IHP+ 2010; DFID 2007).

The opportunities to use targeted resources to maximize the provision of a wider package of health interventions have generally not been realized. New terminologies have emerged, including the concept of a "diagonal" approach or "campaign vertically, spend horizontally." Proponents argue that resources earmarked for a particular disease, such as HIV/AIDS, can serve to spearhead improvements in health systems (WHO 2007a).

A number of formal international commitments have centered around improved coordination, alignment behind nationally led plans, and efforts to make development assistance more predictable and sustainable (OECD 2005) across all sectors as well as in health, in particular (DFID 2007). At the launch of the International Health Partnership in 2007, the U.K. government described the health environment—with 40 bilateral donors, 90 global health initiatives, 26 UN agencies, and 20 global and regional funds—as being overly complex (DFID 2007).

In 2008, the High-level Taskforce on Innovative Financing for Health Systems reviewed the constraints on health systems, the costs of scaling up health care, possible sources of additional finance, and options to channel such funding. It explored opportunities to make aid more predictable and better linked to results. From this process emerged a "common health systems funding platform" for the GFATM, GAVI, and the World Bank, the largest providers of support for health systems development. It accepted that the major investments in HIV/AIDS, tuberculosis, malaria, and childhood vaccination and maternal health are constrained by the quality of the underlying health system, recognized the fragmented and disorganized state of development assistance for health, and stressed the need for an improved relationship between disease-focused programs and the development of comprehensive health systems. The common platform is intended to support a single country plan and budget as well as a single implementation process and results framework. It builds upon the Paris Declaration and Accra Principles on aid effectiveness and the International Health Partnership (DFID 2007). The platform will be performance based and take an incremental approach to reducing bottlenecks to service delivery, reducing transaction costs, and rationalizing the number of duplicative initiatives in the health sector. However, in 2010, it is difficult to see any progress by individual organizations in balancing their agendas with the needs of countries.

The importance of coordination and accountability is heighted by the narrow focus of many global health initiatives and the growing adoption of output-based performance measures that may inadvertently encourage targeting at the expense of wider systems strengthening. The continuing competition for public attention and funding as well as the emphasis on short-term "deliverables" may undermine efforts to ensure a more organized system of mutual accountability, coordination, and partnership (Buse and Harmer 2007).

Implementation of the Paris Principles has met with limited success. A 2008 review by the OECD found that many donors still insist on using their own parallel fiduciary systems, even in countries that have good-quality systems. This review reported on 14,000 donor missions that were conducted in 54 recipient countries in one year, with Vietnam fielding an average of three per day (OECD 2008b).

In 2003, Unger et al. (2003) proposed a code of best practice for disease control to avoid damaging health care services in developing countries. They recognized that these programs only meet a fraction of demand or need for health care, contributing to inefficient facility use by recipients and gaps in care. External funding can undermine government capacity by reducing the responsibility of the state to improve its own services. Unger et al. concluded that most, but not all, vertical disease programs should be integrated into general health service delivery, and that their administration and operations should be designed with reference to existing systems and planned to integrate into these rather than establish new systems. They emphasized the need to avoid conflict with health care delivery, including advance planning for potential damage control.

In addition, Garrett (2007) highlights the dangers in the continuing lack of coordination, competition among providers, and the disproportionate sums directed at specific high-profile diseases rather than in improving public health in general. While substantial aid is tied to meeting narrow disease targets, critical systemic needs (including the world shortage of four million health workers) remain largely unmet.

For diseases of poverty (i.e., largely communicable diseases), Buse and Harmer (2007) identify the positive contributions that global health initiatives have made by:

- helping specific health issues get on national and international agendas,
- mobilizing additional resources,
- stimulating research and development,

- improving access to cost-effective health interventions among populations with limited ability to pay,
- strengthening national health policy processes and content, and
- augmenting service delivery capacity and establishing international norms and standards.

However, they also highlight habits that result in suboptimal performance and negative externalities:

- skewing national priorities by imposing external ones,
- depriving specific stakeholders a voice in decision making,
- inadequate governance practices,
- misguided assumptions on the efficiency of the public and private sectors,
- insufficient resources to implement partnership activities and costs,
- wasting resources through inadequate use of country systems, and
- poor harmonization and inappropriate incentives for health care staff.

Fragile Health Systems

Health systems that are too fragile and fragmented to deliver the volume and quality of services to those in need constitute a primary bottleneck to achieving the Millennium Development Goals in low-income countries. The World Health Report 2000 described a health system as "all the activities [including all organizations, institutions, resources, people and activities] whose primary purpose is to promote, restore or maintain health" (WHO 2000b:5) and outlined four essential functions: service provision, resource generation, financing, and stewardship. In 2006, WHO defined health systems strengthening as "building capacity in critical components of health systems to achieve more equitable and sustained improvements across health services and health outcomes" (WHO 2006b:10). In practical terms, this means addressing the key systemic constraints related to the health workforce, infrastructure, health commodities (e.g., equipment and medicines), logistics and supply, tracking progress, and effective financing necessary to provide services that are responsive to need and financially fair. There is an overwhelming need to address the perception that health systems are complex, to demystify the health systems strengthening agenda, and to improve governance and strategic planning that underpin performance. Two areas of the "health systems agenda" warrant particular attention: the complex financing of health and the global health workforce crisis.

Global health funding increased from USD 2.5 billion in 1990 to almost USD 14 billion in 2005 (World Bank 2007). In addition to the increase in official development assistance, private funding for global health now accounts for a quarter of all health development aid (Bloom 2007). The increasing number of global health actors has made tracking global health funding increasingly difficult. McCoy and colleagues (2009) highlight the complexity and fragmentation of global health financing and inadequate monitoring and tracking. The proliferation of actors and the convoluted financing channels lead to substantial transaction costs and greater difficulty in ensuring accountability to the public. The World Bank has stated that "unless deficiencies in the global aid architecture are corrected and major reforms occur at the country level, the international community and countries themselves face a good chance of squandering" the rise in attention and money directed at improving the health of the world's poor (World Bank 2007:149).

There are concerns that "substitution" through increased international aid leads to reductions in government funding for health. Lu et al. (2010) showed that for every dollar of aid, government funding falls by USD 0.43–1.14. Ooms et al. (2010) propose that governments compensate for exceptional international generosity to the health sector by reallocating government funding to other sectors, that they anticipate the unreliability of international health aid over the long term by stalling increases in recurrent health expenditure, or that they smooth aid by spreading it across several years. International assistance for health is generally unpredictable and poorly suited to fund recurrent costs.

A second major systems challenge is the health workforce crisis attributable to a combination of circumstances: inadequate production, poor salaries and working conditions, increased migration, and losses through AIDS. The Joint Learning Initiative (JLI) initiated by the Rockefeller Foundation, the World Health Report in 2006, and the creation of the Global Health Workforce Alliance in 2006 raised the profile and scale of the problem and helped to build consensus on possible effective responses (Rockefeller Foundation 2003; WHO 2006b). The JLI Working Group on Priority Diseases highlighted the impact of a substantial number of global health initiatives in developing countries.

Until recently, the donor community has been reluctant to provide the necessary structural support to the health workforce beyond the funding of short training courses. Important donors, such as the Bill & Melinda Gates Foundation (BMGF) and GFATM, have been very restrictive despite the recognition that the successful implementation of initiatives is severely hampered by workforce limitations. A trained workforce is at the core of the health system. A typical country devotes just over 42% of total government health expenditure to pay for its health workforce, though there are regional and country variations. In Africa, 3% of the global health workforce struggles to manage 24% of the burden of disease (WHO 2006e). Low-income countries face common challenges: how to effect a rapid increase in the number of appropriately skilled and motivated health service providers and ensure that they are equitably distributed; how to maximize the productivity of the workforce; and how to motivate health workers to stay and serve their communities and reduce losses.

Mounting evidence indicates that the following approaches have yielded success:

- shift tasks to lower skilled workers,
- change the skills mix of the workforce,
- expand and increase the capabilities of cadres of community-based workers, and
- influence staff distribution through targeted use of incentives.

Support for health workforce planning and management information systems has slowly increased, as have efforts to improve productivity (WHO 2006e).

Elimination/eradication initiatives have attracted "philanthropic volunteers" to raise funds and support activities (e.g., immunization days for polio and measles, mass drug distribution campaigns against NTDs). Building on the success of community-directed treatment in reaching remote populations, the African Program for Onchocerciasis Control (APOC) studied the potential to use this approach to deliver other interventions and had considerable success in delivering malaria treatment, insecticide-treated mosquito nets, and vitamin A (UNICEF et al. 2008). Many other health and nonhealth programs also make extensive use of volunteers, and thus opportunities exist for greater coordination around training, sequencing of activities, and harmonizing incentives across initiatives.

The U.S. Global Health Act of 2010 is a response to the recognition that health systems in many low-income countries are broken. It includes a new global health workforce initiative to support a comprehensive approach meeting health workforce needs. This is part of a wider global health initiative, which promises a radical change in the development model of the United States, the largest donor, with a possible move from a targeted approach to one that aims to better coordinate efforts across the U.S. Government and with other donors and contribute to the development of sustainable health systems (U.S. Global Health Initiative 2010).

How Have Disease Eradication Programs Affected Health Systems?

Each eradication initiative has provided lessons to inform future efforts (Henderson 1998; Taylor et al. 1997; Aylward et al. 2000a; Hopkins, this volume). The next generation of elimination/eradication initiatives will look for guidance from the Global Polio Eradication Initiative (GPEI; see Aylward, this volume), and perhaps to the measles elimination initiative (see Andrus et al., this volume). Elimination/eradication initiatives offer major opportunities to improve coordination among partners, dialog across countries, and the realization of wider health benefits, but these opportunities have not been fully exploited.

More recent elimination efforts, such as those against NTDs, have demonstrated considerable awareness of the wider health systems challenges and have increasingly adopted an integrated approach linked with other programs (Gyapong et al. 2010). There are indications that the large budget global health initiatives, such as GAVI and GFATM, are following this path.

GPEI has helped generate substantial, additional resources and commitment from groups such as Rotary International. NTD elimination programs have attracted significant in-kind donations of drugs from the pharmaceutical industry. However, while most financial resources have been provided through external partners, elimination/eradication initiatives incur substantial local costs, and these have been poorly quantified.

In its review of the expanded program of immunization and early polio eradication initiatives in Latin America, the Taylor Commission concluded that the program delivered mixed effects and missed opportunities (Taylor et al. 1995). It highlighted the need for implementation to be part of a systemic program to build health infrastructure. Substantial benefits were, however, evident: There was cooperation across sectors and improved links between health workers and communities. The initiatives also generated pride in national achievement, raised the profile of health, and fostered intercountry collaboration, even across war zones. Management capacity was strengthened, and donors directly funded districts for the first time. The coordinating mechanisms established were used to manage other disease epidemics, and there was some co-delivery of other interventions (e.g., micronutrients). There was cooperation across laboratories and enhanced disease surveillance in the Americas. However, Taylor et al. (1995) cautioned that the benefits could only be applied to countries with established and sustainable health systems, strong leadership at central and district levels, a well-organized infrastructure, and local ownership and decision making. They warned against generalizing findings from more-developed to less-developed regions of the world, and described negative effects of global immunization goals that were in conflict with local demands and priorities, an issue also reported in relation to polio eradication in Nigeria. Training was often described as disrupting services and diverting the workforce from regular tasks. There was often little coordination with other priority programs, and most training was through in-service courses rather than through early adaptation of basic curricula. Their literature review highlighted the dearth of documentation on lessons learned to guide best practice. This situation continues today with the failure to view the collective impact of many such targeted programs on the health sector.

In 1997, concern was raised on ethical dilemmas related to polio eradication (Taylor et al. 1997). The balance of global goals and local priorities was put into question: Should poor countries, which have many priority health problems that are controllable using the available low cost-effective interventions, divert limited resources to pursue a global goal that has perhaps lower priority for their own children? Taylor et al. (1997) raised concerns about promoting

1. An eradication initiative needs to be based on technically sound strategies with proven operational feasibility in a large geographical area.
2. An informed collective decision needs to be negotiated by an appropriate international forum to minimize long-term risks in financing and implementation.
3. Sufficient resources need to be deployed at the community level in a partnership.
4. Appropriate financing strategies are vital.
5. At the outset, those countries or populations likely to delay achievement of the global goal must be identified to ensure provision of sufficient resources and attention.
6. International health goals, such as polio eradication, must be designed and pursued within existing health systems if they are to secure and sustain broad support.

The evaluation of the impact of an eradication initiative on health systems has been hampered by the lack of baseline data, the absence of control groups, and the concurrent implementation of major health reforms.

While the elimination/eradication model is time limited, GPEI demonstrates that the time frame can extend to the point where doubts are raised on the feasibility of eradication. The endorsement of global goals by the WHA in 1988 may not be translated into prioritization in country health programs and budgets over many years, and in light of continuing and new challenges to the health of the population and the advent of new well-funded global health initiatives.

How Can Future Elimination/Eradication Initiatives Best Contribute to the Strengthening of Health Systems?

The WHO resolution that launched the GPEI stated that eradication should be pursued in ways that strengthened the delivery of specific health services or the development of health systems (WHO 1988). Although there is no shortage of advice for future elimination/eradication initiatives in terms of methodology, there is little evidence on how to apply that guidance. Melgaard et al. (1998) set out a framework for the design of future eradication programs to ensure the greatest benefit accrues to health systems development. Aylward et al. (2003) has highlighted key lessons from past programs. Key recommendations to guide interactions between global health initiative and country health systems have been delineated by the World Health Organization Maximizing Positive Synergies Collaborative Group (2009).

Perhaps it is appropriate to first question whether elimination/eradication initiatives can contribute to health systems strengthening or whether, because of their very nature, they are in conflict with long-term systems building.

Can initiatives that promote globally defined health priorities, as determined by international institutions, effectively engage with and support national governments, which seek to deliver universal access to services specific to the priority health needs of their populations?

The global health environment of 2010 looks very different from that of the 1970s or 1980s, when the current generation of elimination/eradication initiatives were conceived. At present, the international- and country-level settings are far more complex: many more stakeholders, small projects, funding, and complex financing channels exist than in earlier decades. This creates many more opportunities to do good, but also the potential for interactions to do harm.

Health priorities will continue to evolve. In all regions except Africa, noncommunicable diseases account for the greatest share of the burden of disease. Climate change is expected to result in uncertain health impacts, and the emergence of newly emerging infectious diseases remains a constant threat.

Viewed in 2010, the Millennium Development Goals are unlikely to be met by 2015, and the post-2015 global development agenda is unclear. Aid priorities and modalities of donors and global health initiatives will continue to evolve, and new actors (e.g., China, India, and Brazil and large multinational corporations) will further influence the development landscape. Earmarking of future aid for globally defined priorities may, as today, not bear a relation to the major causes of the burden of disease in a country.

The debate on the merits of vertical and horizontal approaches will continue. Countries will likely continue to pursue a pragmatic mix of approaches that blend targeted, disease- or intervention-specific and horizontal, health system-strengthening strategies. They will likely continue to struggle to achieve the right mix and maximum benefits.

Underfunded and dysfunctional health systems, fragile political alliances, disruptions through conflict, weak governance and communities with little faith in government will likely continue to be the norm in the poorest countries. National health and development budgets in the poorest countries will remain stretched despite increased aid.

Sustaining hard won gains will be a challenge. History suggests that the recent high levels of investment in health are unlikely to continue with many other development priorities (e.g., economic growth, food and water security) demanding attention. Over recent decades, donor support for malaria and immunization has varied widely as new funds have been allocated to new challenges. The introduction of new, more expensive vaccines, initially subsidized by GAVI, will increase pressure on national budgets. GAVI has not yet achieved downward price leverage on new vaccines to the degree expected, and the global economic downturn may limit the level of ambition and the acceptance of relatively high cost vaccines.

Future elimination/eradication initiatives must balance their specific goals against the common threats to health and life in the poorest countries. They need to deliver short-term gains (results) while maximizing opportunities to co-deliver a range of interventions (efficiency) and build a health service over the longer term (sustainability)—one that is able to respond to the current and future needs of populations. When GPEI was launched, the major health challenges that children faced in low-income countries were pneumonia, diarrhea, measles, malaria, and malnutrition. With the addition of HIV/AIDS, these remain largely unchanged today.

In addition to meeting time-bound disease reduction targets, elimination/eradication initiatives will need to respond better to aid effectiveness challenges and maximize investment in national capacity and the wider health system. This implies alignment behind the national development plan, support for meaningful country ownership, and the division of labor with others. Initiatives will thus need to consider the predictability of finance, minimize transaction costs, and ensure that their efforts complement those of other priority interventions to reduce duplication and overlap.

At the outset, an initiative must understand the country context within which it will operate, including the policy environment and national priorities, the complex financing flows, the challenges that governments face in managing multiple stakeholders, and the gaps in a country's ability to carry out essential public health functions. Of particular importance are approaches to disease surveillance, health education and information, monitoring and evaluation, workforce development, enforcement of public health laws and regulations and public health research. Each initiative should carry out a health system impact assessment in advance of operations and judge their contribution to the collective impact of many such targeted programs on the health sector. The reversals in polio suggest that advance management of damage control should be part of the planning process.

Future elimination/eradication initiatives need to be placed from the outset in a long-term framework designed to strengthen health systems, one in which there is a clear fit with the national health strategy and in a way that offers maximum benefits to systems strengthening without jeopardizing eradication achievements. Wherever possible, initiatives should work through and build upon existing systems of planning and management, logistics and supply, finance, and information. They should actively seek co-delivery of other health interventions using a range of platforms inside and outside the formal health system. It will be important to maximize planning and implementation links with partners at the country and international level that target diseases/interventions (GAVI, GFATM) and those that address systematic bottlenecks (GHWA, Health Metrics Network). Greater focus needs to be placed on building the capacity of routine systems (immunization, surveillance, service delivery) in the weakest environments from the onset.

In 2010, a major candidate for eradication is measles (WHO 2010a), which will build on long, if intermittent, investment in improving routine immunization systems to achieve high levels of national coverage. Supplementary immunization activities, however, cannot replace the lack of routine services. Investments in improving surveillance and laboratory capacity are being designed to provide the widest possible benefits from the start and complement investments from other targeted programs, such as the Health Metrics Network (health information) and HIV/AIDS and NTD programs (laboratories). The experiences from universal childhood immunization programs and GPEI provide lessons on how to ensure that synergies are maximized and to strengthen delivery of health services in the poorest districts of countries.

Elimination/eradication initiatives should set targets and indicators to measure their impact and performance against key points of interaction with the health system: service delivery, financing, governance, health workforce, health information, and supply management. WHO developed such a framework for optimizing the impact of polio activities on expanded immunization programs, although this was not fully implemented (WHO 2001a), and the International Health Partnership (DFID 2007) developed a set of health systems indicators as part of a common monitoring and evaluation framework.

The polio experience demonstrates that the initial global endorsement of an eradication goal may not translate into country plans and budgets over decades. Thus, there will need to be continued investment in advocacy at the global and country level. The best way to maintain support over the long term, particularly at the community level, may be through demonstrating the positive impact of the elimination/eradication initiative on the provision of wider services and the overall health system.

It is important to temper disease- or intervention-specific advocacy with recognition of the dangers of narrow earmarking, which may undermine wider health objectives. Wherever possible, investment should be made in systematic improvements using targeted funds to build and strengthen existing systems.

Future elimination/eradication initiatives must also invest in building evidence early. The WHO Maximizing Positive Synergies Collaborative Group (2009) makes a number of recommendations that are applicable to elimination/eradication initiatives as well as to the studied global health initiatives. These include the need to:

- Infuse the health systems strengthening agenda with the same sense of ambition and speed that has characterized the global health initiatives.
- Extend the health remit of narrowly focused global health initiatives and agree to indicators for health systems strengthening.
- Improve the alignment of planning processes and resource allocations among global health initiatives as well as between global health initiatives and country health systems.
- Generate more reliable data for the costs and benefits of strengthening health systems and evidence to inform additional and complementary investments to those of global health initiatives.

- Ensure a rise in national and global health financing and in more predictable financing to support the sustainable and equitable growth of health systems.

Conclusion

Disease eradication and elimination initiatives will continue to be a part of the development landscape but need to demonstrate compatibility with health care planning, financing, and delivery in poor countries. They need to contribute to efforts to build health systems and should unite the delivery of short-term, discrete targets against individual diseases with investment in building the capacity of health services to deliver universal, affordable access to care. Deliberate policy decisions are needed at the onset of new disease elimination/eradication initiatives. The evidence and arguments set out in this chapter should help in this task.

Acknowledgments

Tim Martineau (Liverpool School of Tropical Medicine), Eve Worrall (Liverpool Associates in Tropical Health), and Robert Steinglass (John Snow International (JSI)) provided helpful comments on the draft.

17

The Impacts of Measles Elimination Activities on Immunization Services and Health Systems in Six Countries

Piya Hanvoravongchai, Sandra Mounier-Jack,
Valeria Oliveira Cruz, Dina Balabanova, Robin Biellik,
Yayehyirad Kitaw, Tracey Koehlmoos, Sebastião Loureiro,
Mitike Molla, Ha Trong Nguyen, Pierre Ongolo-Zogo,
Umeda Sadykova, Harbandhu Sarma, Maria Gloria Teixeira,
Jasim Uddin, Alya Dabbagh, and Ulla Kou Griffiths

Abstract

Measles is a prime candidate for global eradication. Explicit goals to control or eliminate the disease have already been agreed upon by many countries and regions. One
of the key concerns in determining the appropriateness of establishing the measles
eradication goal is its potential impact on routine immunization services and the overall health system. To evaluate the impact of accelerated measles elimination activities
(AMEAs) on immunization services and health systems, a study was conducted in six
countries: Bangladesh, Brazil, Cameroon, Ethiopia, Tajikistan, and Vietnam. Primary
data were collected through key informant interviews and staff profiling surveys. Secondary data were obtained from policy documents, studies, and reports. Data analysis
used mainly qualitative approaches.

The study found that the impact of AMEAs varied, with positive and negative implications in specific immunization and health system functions. On balance, the impacts on immunization services were largely positive in all six countries, particularly
in Bangladesh, Brazil, Tajikistan, and Vietnam; negative impacts were more significant
in Cameroon and Ethiopia. Although weaker health systems may not be able to benefit sufficiently from AMEAs, in more developed health systems, disruption to health
service delivery is unlikely to occur. Nevertheless, in none of the six countries was
there an explicit objective to use AMEAs to help remove health system bottlenecks and

strengthen system capacity. Opportunities to strengthen routine immunization services and the health system should be actively sought to address system's bottlenecks so that benefits from the measles eradication activities as well as other health priorities can be optimized.

Introduction

Measles is the prime target as the next disease for a global eradication campaign. Its biological characteristics and effective intervention make it a feasible disease to eradicate at the current point in time (de Quadros et al. 2008). Considerable progress has already been achieved toward the global goal of a 90% reduction in measles mortality by 2010 (Dabbagh et al. 2009). In fact, five of the six WHO regions have already adopted a measles elimination target. Consequently, at the 2010 World Health Assembly, milestones toward measles eradication were endorsed (WHO 2010a).

One of the key concerns in determining the appropriateness of measles eradication is its potential impact on routine immunization services and the overall health system. Experiences from previous eradication efforts have shown that eradication activities tend to be conducted using a vertical approach, due to their targeted and time-limited nature. The debate around vertical versus horizontal modes of delivery has long been part of the public health literature (Bradley 1998; Cairncross et al. 1997; Frenk 2006; Mills 1983; Walsh and Warren 1979). Whereas some authors take the view that a horizontal or more integrated approach is preferable, since it includes contributions from other sectors and is more sustainable (Rifkin and Walt 1986), others argue that a more selective or vertical approach is required in view of resource constraints (Walsh and Warren 1979).

There are also questions on potential synergies between priority disease programs and the health systems, and how these disease programs can contribute to health systems strengthening. Although many reasons have contributed to the delays in achieving the eradication targets for guinea worm and poliomyelitis, one common factor is that residual transmissions take place in countries with extremely weak health systems (Wakabi 2009; Wassilak and Orenstein 2010). According to an independent evaluation of the polio eradication initiative, this program needs to contribute more systematically to immunization systems strengthening if interruption of the virus is to be accomplished in the remaining endemic countries (Mohamed et al. 2009; Global Polio Eradication Initiative 2010). With the substantial increase in the aid volume to combat diseases in developing countries, the debate on priority diseases and health systems has gained new momentum, and the term "diagonal" approach has been coined to argue that resources earmarked for a particular disease (e.g., HIV/AIDS) can serve to spearhead improvements in health systems (Atun et al. 2010; Ravishankar et al. 2009).

Table 17.2   Most recent supplementary immunization activities (SIAs) for measles in the six study countries.

Country	Year	Target population	Type	Vaccine used	Interventions included in SIAs
Bangladesh	2010	20,000,000	Follow-up	Measles	Vitamin A and polio vaccine
Brazil	2008	69,700,000	Catch-up	MMR	Catch-up EPI vaccines, health education on dental care, hypertension, diabetes, and STDs
Cameroon	2009	3,435,546	Follow-up	Measles	Vitamin A, polio vaccine, catch-up EPI vaccines including TT for women, IPTp, anti-helminthics[1], yellow fever vaccine in selected districts
Ethiopia	2009	276,695	Follow-up	Measles	Vitamin A and anti-helminthics[1]
Tajikistan	2009	2,340,440	Catch-up	MR	Vitamin A and mebendazole[1]
Vietnam	2009	1,036,222	Subnational follow-up	Measles	Vitamin A

[1]   Mebendazole or albendazole for deworming

MMR: measles–mumps–rubella combined vaccine; EPI: expanded program on immunization; STDs: sexually transmitted diseases; TT: tetanus toxoid vaccine; IPTp: intermittent preventive treatment in pregnancy; MR: measles–rubella combined vaccine

- *Vietnam* introduced a nationwide routine second dose in 2006 for all first-grade children at the time of school entry. Its latest subnational follow-up SIA took place in five provinces in 2008 and reached a target population of over a million individuals between the ages of 7–20.

Integration of Measles Activities into the EPI and Health System

Within Routine EPIs

While measles vaccination was reported to be, in general, fully integrated within routine EPI programs in all countries, SIAs were implemented in a less integrated manner within routine EPI programs, dependent on a number of EPI functions. In terms of financing, for example, SIAs tended to attract a high proportion of external funds that needed to be used independently of other EPI activities in all countries except Brazil and Vietnam. For planning, SIAs required specific planning exercises in most countries. In addition, the information system for SIAs often required dedicated reporting forms that were adapted or developed from routine reporting forms, such as in Ethiopia, to accommodate reporting of additional public health interventions delivered during SIAs.

Integration of EPIs within the Health System

In most countries, with the exception of Brazil and to some extent Bangladesh, EPIs generally operated as a vertical program; they had their own funding stream, dedicated staff at the national level, specific procurement and logistics systems, and separate planning and information system. Brazil had by far the most integrated system; all EPI functions operated as routine health services. In the other countries, certain EPI functions were less integrated into the wider health system (e.g., financing, logistics, and health information). Logistics tended to be managed separately from other supply chains within the Ministries of Health, and procurement was often carried out by the UNICEF procurement facility. In many cases, this separation stems from historical patterns of government funding and donor investment. The information system in Vietnam was not integrated; separate reporting forms were used for specific vaccine-preventable diseases.

Service delivery and disease surveillance are the EPI functions that were most integrated into health systems. At the service-delivery level, vaccination services were, to a large extent, well integrated with primary care services; they were delivered by general or multipurpose health workers, although they retained a vertical element when vaccinations were offered through dedicated outreach services. Across all study countries, vaccine-preventable disease surveillance accounted for one of the most integrated health functions, notably owing to the integrated disease surveillance system which shares resources and data collection as well as reporting and laboratory diagnostic procedures across several diseases.

Governance of EPIs was more difficult to assess. Some countries have a high degree of integration with mother and child health (MCH) teams, as in Ethiopia and Bangladesh, whereas elsewhere it was independent from other programs and had limited contact with other departments. Governance of the EPI program tended to be less integrated within the health system at higher levels, while being more integrated at district level or below. This was also the case for overall planning. In Tajikistan, however, staff involved in conducting routine measles activities had limited formal collaboration with family doctors, whose role it is to organize primary health care in a specific area, or with MCH staff. Vaccination services in Tajikistan were seen as separate from the rest of primary care activities: a system inherited from the Soviet model prior to independence in 1991.

Table 17.3 summarizes the integration of EPI within the health system and AMEAs within the EPI for all six countries.

Table 17.3 Integrating measles activities with EPI and health systems.

	Cameroon		Ethiopia		Tajikistan		Vietnam		Bangladesh		Brazil[1]
	EPI and health system	Measles SIAs and EPI	EPI and health system	Measles SIAs and EPI	EPI and health system	Measles SIAs and EPI	EPI and health system	Measles SIAs and EPI	EPI and health system	Measles SIAs and EPI	EPI and health system
Governance	Linkage	Coordination	Linkage	Coordination	Linkage	Coordination	Full integration	Full integration	Full integration	Full integration	Full integration
Financing	Linkage	No interaction	Linkage	No interaction	No interaction	No interaction	Linkage	Coordination	Coordination	Coordination	Full integration
Planning	Linkage	Coordination	Coordination	Coordination	Linkage	Coordination	Linkage	Coordination	Full integration	Full integration	Full integration
Human resources	Coordination	Coordination	Coordination	Coordination	Full integration	Coordination	Linkage	Full integration	Full integration	Full integration	Full integration
Logistics	No interaction	Coordination	No interaction	Coordination	No interaction	Coordination	Coordination	Full integration	No interaction	Full integration	Full integration
Information system	Linkage	Coordination	No interaction	Coordination	Linkage	Full integration	Full integration	Full integration	Linkage	Full integration	Full integration
Surveillance	Linkage	Full integration	Coordination	Full integration	No interaction	Full integration	Full integration	Full integration	Full integration	Full integration	Full integration
Service delivery	Coordination	Coordination	Coordination	Coordination	Full integration	Full integration	Full integration	Linkage	Full integration	Full integration	Full integration

[1] Not enough information available to analyze the level of integration of measles SIAs and EPI in Brazil

Full integration: the majority of the program elements are fully integrated.

Coordination: most elements share common strategies, policies, or activities with the system, or there is a balance mixture of integrated and nonintegrated elements.

Linkage: some interactions between the program and the system exist, but there are no coordinated activities.

No interaction: the majority of the program elements have no formal interactions and is thus not integrated into the system.

Impacts of AMEAs on Immunization Services and Health System

The impacts of AMEAs were assessed according to each of the eight components: governance, planning and management, financing, human resources, logistics and procurement, information system, surveillance, and service delivery and demand generation. A summary of the results is provided by function below, with accompanying statements from some informants.

Governance

According to key informants in all countries, AMEAs contributed to partnership building across Ministry of Health departments and stimulated collaboration across partner agencies to improve EPI governance and service delivery. In Bangladesh, Ethiopia, and Tajikistan, open involvement of communities and community leaders improved the accountability of EPI and raised awareness about the importance of immunization at both national and local levels. In Cameroon, Vietnam, Bangladesh, and Tajikistan, measles SIAs fostered active involvement from political leaders.

> According to a health staff member in Vietnam: "The success of measles campaigns can be used as the most persuasive evidence to lobby for preventive medicine."

> A district hospital physician in Tajikistan reported that "after the SIAs, local authorities are more attentive and responsive to child health care issues."

However, some key informants in Cameroon and Ethiopia expressed concerns over the imposition of funding conditions and the use of SIAs as the main elimination strategy. Donor earmarking of funding for measles activities was perceived as undermining local resource allocation decisions. Informants also believed that the implementation of measles SIAs as a priority activity separate from general health system strategies contributed to fragmented policy-making and priority-setting. In Ethiopia and Tajikistan, measles SIAs were perceived by some to have reduced motivation for adequate investment in broader health service delivery and primary health care.

Planning and Management

AMEAs helped to develop strategies and skills required for planning and management at all government levels and stimulated interdepartmental and intersectoral planning. This was particularly the case in Cameroon and Ethiopia, which used the opportunity of annual Child Health Days to deliver measles vaccines, and involved the complex planning of multiple child health-related interventions. Strengthened skills included the capacity to identify, map, and target hard-to-reach populations, both for vaccination and other outreach activities. In Ethiopia, preparations for SIAs required the development of innovative strategies to cover the underdeveloped Afar and Somali regions. In Tajikistan, SIAs achieved high coverage among groups that are traditionally isolated geographically for parts of the year.

> From a health staff member in Vietnam: "My skills for planning and management improved after being trained to do measles SIAs, and it is beneficial for planning and managing other health programs in my commune."

Management skills acquired in the process of implementing measles activities were reported to be applicable to other preventive activities, such as planning for pandemic influenza vaccination. Key informants in Bangladesh and Tajikistan mentioned the stimulation of a culture of long-term planning in the health sector as another positive impact. However, in Cameroon, informants reported that measles SIAs could interfere with planning of routine EPI activities and other health services at regional and district levels. This is mainly because of short notice from the national level with many SIAs being conducted each year for various diseases.

> According to a district informant in Cameroon: "We must stop everything at once to produce results....activities that were planned in March had to be shifted to April because of SIAs."

> A Cameroon health facility staff reported "If we knew at the beginning of the year when the campaign would take place, we would be able to solve many issues."

Financing

Findings from key informant interviews show mixed patterns of impact that AMEAs had on the financing of immunization services, in particular, and health systems, in general. In all countries except Brazil, measles elimination activities helped leverage additional fund-raising from local and international partners to deliver both measles activities and additional public health interventions. In Bangladesh, Tajikistan, and Vietnam, reports also show that skills in fund raising were enhanced.

At the same time, concern was also expressed that the motivation to strengthen routine immunization services and the health system, in general, could be reduced because external funds were channeled primarily to finance SIAs for measles rather than routine vaccination services. Earmarking of donor funding for SIAs was perceived in Cameroon to be possibly detrimental to longer-term investment in routine vaccination services. However, quantitative evidence from budget allocations failed to show a decrease in resources for non-measles EPI funding in any of the countries. While external partners almost fully funded the Bangladesh catch-up SIAs in 2005–2006, the Bangladesh government largely funded the catch-up SIAs in 2010. In Cameroon, external partners were responsible for financing the procurement of vaccines and delivery of vaccines and integrated interventions during SIAs. In Bangladesh and Vietnam, tensions were reported regarding financing at the district and provincial levels to cover the operational costs of SIAs.

> An informant from Bangladesh stated: "A Civil Surgeon had to ask local health officers to manage money for organizing the SIAs from their own sources as funds from headquarters were delayed."

Human Resources

In many countries, the quantity and quality of EPI staff reportedly increased as a result of AMEAs. Staff size increased, although most were volunteers (e.g., youth and women's groups) who were mobilized for measles SIAs or used to help out in other EPI activities (e.g., temporary or retired staff workers). In regard to quality, key informants in all countries stated that the additional staff training provided as part of preparations for AMEAs helped improve the knowledge and skills of health staff on immunization planning, management, and service delivery as well as disease surveillance, laboratory diagnosis, and information management. In Brazil, skills in vaccine-preventable disease surveillance were especially noted to have improved as a result of AMEAs.

> From a staff member at a Vietnam commune health center: "Yes, knowledge and skills of my commune health center staff on reporting, injection technique, campaign planning, and community mobilization have improved a lot."

The use of incentives and different remuneration mechanisms for staff engaged in measles-related activities produced mixed results. The level of SIA payments, when compared to salary, was low in Vietnam, Bangladesh, and Tajikistan, but could be as high as half of salary income or more for some involved personnel in Cameroon and Ethiopia (Table 17.4). Key informants in Bangladesh and Ethiopia reported that the incentives provided by AMEAs helped motivate staff to become more committed to their responsibilities. In Ethiopia, where additional remuneration provided for SIAs was considerably higher than the government allowance, incentives reportedly contributed to retaining health workers in the public sector. However, negative impacts on other staff not directly involved in AMEAs were also reported. In Cameroon and Tajikistan, some key informants stated that staff may have been less motivated to perform routine immunization activities and other primary care tasks because of the lack of incentives for routine activities.

There were reports of EPI staff feeling overloaded from additional work from SIAs in Bangladesh, Cameroon, Ethiopia, and Vietnam. Results from the staff profiling surveys in Bangladesh, Cameroon, and Ethiopia show that more than two-thirds of the surveyed staff reported skipping other important tasks because of SIAs (Table 17.5).

A Cameroon health facility staff reported: "I was alone during the campaign [to carry out all other activities]."

From a health worker working for a nongovernmental organization: "We are a poor country…if you go to some areas you can find only one or two health workers providing clinical services so what do you do? How can you conduct these [measles] campaigns unless you use these workers?

In Brazil, measles SIAs were only conducted during the weekends with participation of community volunteers; this helped to avoid interruptions to routine

Table 17.4   Survey results on the time required for measles SIAs and estimated remuneration. N/A: not available.

Country[1]	No. of respondents	Range of number of days spent on measles SIAs/campaigns (average number)			Estimated SIA remuneration as % of monthly salary (average)
		Planning	Implementation	Evaluation	
Bangladesh	60	2–42 (13.33)	1–30 (10.9)	N/A	16%
Cameroon	16	2–21 (6.31)	3–10 (6.13)	0–4 (2.19)	6–360% (43%)
Ethiopia	36	1–20 (5.6)	3–30 (9.8)	0–4 (1)	36–562% (157%)
Tajikistan	25	30–180 (73)	15 (15)	0–20 (12)	0–91% (35%)
Vietnam	351	1–15 (7.02)	2–12 (2.52)	N/A	Less than 10%

[1]   Staff profiling surveys were not conducted in Brazil because measles elimination had already been achieved.

Table 17.5   Survey results on staff's opinion regarding the impacts of measles SIAs. N/A: not available

Country[1]	No. of respondents	Skip important tasks because of campaign	Believe measles SIAs slow down routine immunization	Believe measles SIAs improve routine immunization	Support a measles elimination goal
Bangladesh	60	86%	0%	83%	87%
Cameroon	16	75%	60%	93%	100%
Ethiopia	36	72%	18%	93%	100%
Tajikistan	25	N/A	24%	100%	100%
Vietnam	60	21%	5%	84%	96%

[1]   Staff profiling surveys were not conducted in Brazil because measles elimination had been already achieved.

services. Key informants in Bangladesh stated that SIAs enhanced the capacity of immunization staff to work under pressure, while in Tajikistan they reportedly became more energized and motivated to work on other EPI activities because of the feeling of achievement developed from expanding vaccination coverage and positive feedback on their work.

Logistics and Procurement

> From a vaccinator in Tajikistan: "During SIAs we received a new refrigerator."

AMEAs were reported to contribute to the improvement of cold-chain system and logistics in all six countries. In Cameroon and Tajikistan, investment in storage and better management of contaminated sharps became useful for services beyond the EPI programs. Logistics-related skills were enhanced and, in Tajikistan, the benefit extended to the drug delivery system, since the skills learned from vaccine management could also be applied to other pharmaceutical products; an increasing share of these tasks were taken over by government services. In Cameroon, however, a substantial share of transportation activities deployed during measles SIAs were rented rather than purchased, so an opportunity to strengthen the routine EPI program after the SIAs was lost.

Information System

One significant positive impact on the national health information system that was an indirect result from AMEAs was better information on target populations. The expansion of or the improvement in birth registration in Bangladesh, Ethiopia, and Vietnam is valuable and can be used for other EPI activities and health programs. In Tajikistan, AMEAs provided an incentive to reconcile differences between census and facility data, and resulted in an agreed upon basis for coverage calculation. In addition, measles SIAs contributed to the mapping of targets and hard-to-reach populations for EPI outreach activities in Cameroon and Tajikistan.

In Ethiopia and Bangladesh, however, national information requirements from SIAs generated many forms to be completed and submitted separately from the routine reporting system, thus generating an additional workload. A similar pattern of duplication occurred in Tajikistan. This, however, resulted primarily from the existing reporting protocol in the general public health system rather than as a result of the SIAs. In Cameroon and Ethiopia, data collected during SIAs were sent directly to national level without adequate utilization at lower levels.

Surveillance

An integral part of AMEAs is a move from population-based to case-based measles surveillance. All countries reported that AMEAs strengthen disease surveillance skills among EPI staff. National surveillance systems benefited through integrated surveillance for a number of vaccine-preventable diseases and other diseases. New laboratory equipment was purchased in Brazil and Vietnam, which was then available for other disease control activities. In Cameroon and Ethiopia, financial incentives provided for reporting measles cases through the Integrated Disease Surveillance Response system and were found to help improve other disease reporting. At the same time, some key informants in Cameroon voiced concerns over the sustainability of current measles surveillance, since it largely depends upon polio eradication program staff.

Service Delivery

A major concern over the impact of AMEAs was on the performance of the routine immunization system. One key assessment is the change in EPI coverage in relation to measles SIAs. At the national level, our study found no pattern of decrease in DPT3 coverage in the years of measles SIAs in any of the six countries (Figure 17.1). According to a report by the Ministry of Health in Vietnam (2006:5), the big reduction in DPT3 coverage in 2002 was due to shortage of vaccine. Latest statistics for 2009, however, show a decline in DPT3 coverage in Ethiopia and Cameroon. At the district level, data on coverage trends in the study districts were not always available, but findings from staff surveys indicate that the impact on routine immunization was perceived to be more positive than negative (Table 17.4).

One commonly reported benefit of AMEAs on immunization services was its capacity to raise community awareness on the benefits of vaccination and primary health care. Resources made available for SIA mobilization through

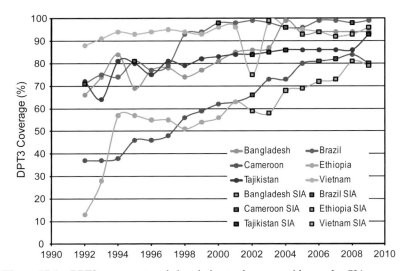

Figure 17.1   DPT3 coverage trends in relation to the years with measles SIAs.

national and local media also reportedly contributed to increased uptake of routine vaccines. It was stated that measles SIAs provided the opportunity to trace and vaccinate defaulters for other vaccines. In Cameroon and Tajikistan, there was an increase in outreach activities to hard-to-reach populations, thus facilitating access to vaccination and other primary care services for these populations. Measles SIAs also stimulated collaboration between state and non-state private providers which resulted in the joint provision of services.

> A national-level key informant in Bangladesh reported: "Before SIAs, we used to visit the people, motivate them to bring their children to the center, but now people themselves mostly come to EPI centers which [has] helped in improving coverage of other vaccines….this is just because of SIAs and publicity."

> A district EPI director in Tajikistan stated that "SIAs help us to reach unreached children."

Although demand for vaccines has increased through social mobilization, in Cameroon, where vaccine-preventable disease SIAs are regularly conducted, concern was expressed that the population might become more passive, possibly waiting for the next campaign rather than actively seeking to complete the routine vaccination schedule.

Because of AMEAs, the quality of immunization service delivery, especially in regard to injection safety and hygiene, has reportedly improved in most countries. Measles SIAs have provided a platform for additional vaccines, including yellow fever, polio, tetanus, BCG, or pentavalent vaccines (Table 17.2). Other public health activities were also included: the delivery of insecticide-treated bed nets, vitamin A supplementation, anti-helminthics, and nutritional screening. It was noted, however, that multiple integrated interventions in SIAs can, in certain circumstances, put pressure on service delivery and be complex to manage.

Effects on other health care services were mixed. In Cameroon and Ethiopia, health care services were interrupted during SIAs because of both staff shortages and inadequate preparation, frequently due to short notice of the event. Some activities at health centers and hospitals were suspended temporarily or only limitedly provided. However, in Bangladesh, key informants stated that health care utilization rates for antenatal care and other primary health care activities had increased due to public mobilization associated with AMEAs. In Tajikistan, there was also an increased demand for primary health care services through social mobilization at local level, which was initially created to support SIAs. Significant reduction in measles outbreaks and morbidity after vaccination also freed up health care facilities in all countries.

> A senior pediatrician in Cameroon: "Most young doctors have never seen a measles case."

Summary of Impacts

Our findings show that the impacts of AMEAs on EPI programs and health systems are highly varied. There are both positive and negative implications in most of the health system and immunization functions. The results also vary with the existing system capacity and context as well as in the way AMEAs were implemented. On balance, positive impacts on immunization service were acknowledged in all countries, particularly Bangladesh, Brazil, Vietnam, and Tajikistan; however, more negative impacts were reported in Cameroon and Ethiopia. Impacts on the health system tend to be limited. A weaker health system may not be able to benefit sufficiently from the AMEAs, whereas in more developed health systems, disruptions are less likely to occur.

Discussion

Earlier studies on polio eradication emphasized potential negative implications for health systems because of resource diversion from routine immunization services and other health programs, particularly in financial and human resources (Aylward and Linkins 2005; Loevinsohn et al. 2002). Our study shows that there is no evidence of a direct financing impact from AMEAs at the national level. This is likely due to the high financial support for vaccines provided by external partners in most countries. Success in measles SIAs was even quoted as bringing credibility to the EPI program to be able to secure more support. However, the earmarking of funds for SIAs by donors was pointed out by several countries as rigid and not conducive to long-term strengthening of routine immunization services. Another reported problem in selected countries was the delay in budget disbursement. In Vietnam there was some tension in funding operational costs that were not provided by the central level.

The possible negative impact on workload and interruption of services was confirmed in this study from both key informant interviews as well as surveys of fieldwork staff. One factor that has contributed to a higher interruption from AMEAs is attributable to the need to mobilize qualified vaccinators for measles vaccine injection; this is not required in polio campaigns. Delays and interruption of health services were reported to vary. Although the period of disruption tends to be short, because SIA implementation did not take long, it was argued that the number of SIAs covering all antigens strained both planning and service delivery, notably in resource-poor countries. Similar to early studies on polio eradication, most of the disruptions could have been avoided through better planning (Aylward and Linkins 2005).

A number of positive impacts on immunization services were found in the country studies. Many of them resulted from having measles activities integrated in the EPI system. Skills of health staff (e.g., immunization service training, program management training) improved and better equipment and information systems (for surveillance, monitoring, and evaluation) were made available, thus benefiting the overall EPI program. By increasing coordination with other sectors, networks were expanded, thus increasing future collaboration on SIAs and mass campaigns for other preventive health programs.

Additional positive impacts beyond immunization occurred when other health care interventions were added to measles SIAs or outreach services, where the existing delivery system was weak. Immunization programs have long been viewed as a natural vehicle for public health interventions and have contributed to increased coverage of the combined interventions, higher efficiency of service delivery, and enhanced equity for multiple interventions in hard-to-reach populations (WHO Regional Office for Africa 2010). It has been argued that key success factors for integration of interventions with SIAs are program compatibility and the existence of a robust EPI program (WHO Regional Office for Africa 2007). We note that in our study, integrated interventions are primarily used in countries where the health system is relatively weak. In Cameroon, as in other countries, coverage achieved for additional interventions was reported to be high (87% coverage rate achieved for deworming in the 2009 measles SIA); however, there were reports that the large number of additional interventions was complex to plan and deliver. Both the number and the effectiveness of integrated interventions in SIAs are rarely evaluated.

Despite our mixed findings on the impacts with mostly positive effects on many functions, particularly on immunization service, the effects were not equally manifested in all six countries. Low-resource countries with weaker underlying systems tend to bear more unfavorable impacts and opportunity costs from AMEAs. In these countries, there could be several disease campaigns each year because of the limited capacity in the routine delivery system, thus creating additional burden on the health care staff, especially when these interventions are not well coordinated and planned. Sustainability of effective service provision is also more at risk when a program's interventions are not effectively integrated into the mainstream of a national health system. Earmarking of funds and separation of logistics or reporting system is not conducive to a long-term strengthening of routine immunization services and health system. Inversely, when the level of integration between AMEAs, routine immunization services, and the health systems is greater, benefits tend to be higher, such as for disease surveillance and health service delivery activities.

Avoiding negative impacts alone is not adequate. Even though eradication initiatives cannot be expected to solve all problems in the health system, it is argued that opportunities to strengthen routine immunization services and health system development need to be actively sought and action taken (Salisbury 1998). Measles eradication strategy should help tackle root causes in the health system that would incur benefits to several priorities simultaneously, thus leveraging the opportunity for success of its program (Travis et al. 2004). In this study, AMEAs were not shown in any of the study countries to have explicit objectives to help strengthen health system capacity beyond improving EPI service and disease surveillance.

The recommendations to include health system strengthening actions with the disease control activities in disease elimination or eradication effort are not new (Taylor and Waldman 1998). Melgaard et al. (1999) recommended that strengthening existing systems should be prioritized over new systems, and donor financing for eradication should be extended to other health system investments. While acknowledging the tensions between the concepts of eradication and sustainable health development, the WHO Workgroup on Disease Elimination/Eradication and Sustainable Health Development made the following recommendation (Salisbury 1998:78):

> Potential benefits of eradication to health development should be identified at the outset …[and] measurable targets should be set for achieving these benefits. The eradication program should be held accountable for the attainment of these wider objectives.

The challenge is how to ensure that these recommendations are translated into actual interventions that are fully financed and included in the disease eradication plans with effective implementation and active monitoring of the impacts. The toolkit developed for this study (Griffiths et al. 2010) can be adapted for country-level impact evaluation assessment.

This study has a number of limitations. Assessing the impact of AMEAs is not conceptually straightforward. Separating the impact of the measles vaccination program from other ongoing immunization efforts is difficult because, in all six countries, AMEAs are integrated to varying degrees in the existing immunization services. In addition, a health system is not static; ongoing changes and reforms complicate the assessment of impact. Nevertheless, efforts were made in all aspects of the study to differentiate the implications of AMEAs from other ongoing activities.

Findings of this study may not be generalizable to a wide range of countries, and there may be inherent bias through selection of informants. However, the case study design sought to employ a range of complementary methods, and efforts have been made to improve the validity of the findings by triangulating data sources and placing data within the context of the existing literature.

Conclusion

This research study in six countries shows that the impacts of measles elimination activities on immunization services and health systems are mixed. There are both positive and negative implications in most of the health system and immunization functions. The results varied with national system capacity and context as well as in the way AMEAs were implemented. The negative implications include perceived diversion of priority from other necessary health interventions, which tend to be more palpable in countries with low resources that rely more on SIAs and a vertical approach to measles elimination. Positive impacts from activities to improve measles vaccination delivery include (a) staff training which leads to improved planning, monitoring and evaluation skills, (b) additional cold-chain and diagnostic laboratory equipment, and (c) better management and information systems which will benefit other EPI activities and primary health care services. On balance, positive impacts on immunization service were acknowledged in all six countries, particularly in Bangladesh, Brazil, Tajikistan, and Vietnam; more negative impacts were reported in Cameroon and Ethiopia. Nevertheless, in none of the six countries were measles eradication activities shown to have an explicit objective to help remove health system bottlenecks and strengthen system capacity.

The study suggests that weaker health systems may not be able to benefit sufficiently from the AMEAs, whereas in more developed systems disruptions are unlikely to occur. The integration of additional services into the planned delivery of measles vaccine could help improve access to health care, especially to those difficult to reach. Potential negative implications regarding EPI programs and health systems must be avoided, and opportunities should be taken to address health system barriers and strengthen routine service delivery to benefit other public health priorities. Obviously, strategies and actions need to be customized specifically to the nature and context of the existing health system in each country as well as to the strategy and activities recommended for measles elimination.

Acknowledgments

Work for completing this paper was granted to LSHTM by the Department of Immunization, Vaccines and Biologicals, World Health Organization. We thank all key informants and survey respondents in the six countries for their participation in this research study. We are thankful to Nicola Lord for her administrative help.

18

Disease Eradication as a Springboard for Broader Public Health Communication

Jeffrey Bates, Sherine Guirguis,
Thomas Moran, and Lieven Desomer

Abstract

In the initial stages of a public health campaign, the mass media is usually very effective in communicating with the majority of the public. Thereafter, focused and intensive engagement is required to reach the underserved, politically, and economically marginalized sectors of society: people who have little social capital, who avoid risks that could destroy the fragile security systems they possess, or those who simply do not have access to the information and services provided to the rest of society. Here is where the final battles against disease are fought. Local initiatives—those which identify the most marginalized segments of society and encourage ownership and participation through intensive interpersonal communication and modifications in service delivery—are necessary to ensure the success of large-scale public health efforts. For all major public health initiatives, the underserved or late adopters are the hardest to reach, yet because an eradication effort must achieve nearly 100% coverage, they hold the key to success or failure. Identifying these groups and understanding the segmentation required even within these minority groups represent critical elements in program design. Strategies and results from the Global Polio Eradication Initiative in India and Nigeria are discussed and applied to the design of future public health and disease eradication initiatives.

Introduction

Health communication has evolved greatly over the past fifty years. Better linkages between social and communication theory, research, and practice have yielded strong evidence for what works best in the field. When communication began to emerge as an area of study, it was guided by claims from the realms of psychology and the social sciences that the mass media could exact immediate and powerful effects. This basic tenet of mass effect informed early health communication efforts and still persists today in many health communication programs. Along with the supposition that mass media could have a dramatic influence on public behavior, the medical establishment widely believed that people, as rational actors, would naturally embrace a behavior that would help them or their loved ones achieve a longer, healthier life.

These assumptions proved wrong. Simple yet obviously beneficial actions (e.g., wearing a safety belt when driving or putting out the cigarette forever) have yet to be universally adopted despite the near universal understanding that such actions are good things to do. Public health officials and communication professionals came to understand that health promotion is very difficult when it involves a lot of people doing something different from what they and their community usually do. Gradually, it was recognized that social identity, cultural norms, and political dynamics all play important roles in whether a person adopts a required behavior, and it is through these social and personal channels that behaviors can be best promoted.

Fortunately for disease control and eradication, most health interventions do not require drastic behavior changes. Social behaviors around health are usually positive, with the majority of the public demanding better and more impactful preventative and curative services. However, people do not always make healthy choices even if they are well aware of the risk and dangers of continuing behavior or not changing their ways. Thus the role of health communication is to interact with communities by providing information and assisting in service delivery so that people can be persuaded to participate in specific health actions.

In the process of adoption, the most difficult phases are the introduction of an innovation, when only risk takers or people with special interests pick up the behavior, and the final stages, when late adopters persistently remain difficult to reach. Late adopters—those who adhere to old practices, take an oppositional perspective to new ways, or are simply out of reach of the health system—pose one of the most significant threats to an eradication initiative, which by definition needs to reach everyone. Whether the public health objective is to get the public to hold out their arm for a single vaccination prick, use a mosquito bed net, or accept multiple doses of oral polio vaccine (OPV) for their children beyond the prescribed immunization schedule, late adopters hold the key to the ultimate success or failure of any eradication effort.

In the initial stages of a public health campaign, mass media is usually very effective at reaching the majority of the public who are the first to adopt an innovation, according to the theory of diffusion of innovations (Rogers 2003). However, the public health world has learned that once you have painted over the public health canvas with the large brush of mass media, there are small pockets that resist or miss out on these broad strokes. These are usually underserved, political and economically marginalized people who have little social capital and avoid risks that could destroy the fragile security systems they already have, or those who simply do not have access to the information and services provided to the rest of society. It is in these pockets that the final battles against the disease are fought. At this phase, when success seems so close and as groups grow to recognize that eradication is high on the state agenda, the nature of the eradication effort itself empowers these groups by giving them leverage to negotiate issues more salient to their needs (Taylor 2009). Local initiatives that encourage ownership and participation, and which complement mass media efforts with intensive interpersonal communication and environmental modifications in service delivery have proven most successful in countering this type of resistance.

A quick look at the public health communication literature tells us that:

- Having a health communication theory in place at the start of the campaign to guide research, implementation, and evaluation increases the chances for success.
- Formative research is essential to understand public sentiment, including both challenges and opportunities, around the health service or behavior.
- Messages have more recall and impact when they are simple, personal, vivid, and repeated messages from multiple sources.
- Audiences are active participants in the communication process; thus health communication efforts need to monitor constantly how messages are interpreted, knowledge and sentiment created, and information shared to keep the campaign on course.

The key lessons to be applied to future eradication efforts, however, are that the pockets of late adopters need to be anticipated in the beginning of the campaign and that from the start, large-scale efforts need to be supplemented by nurturing the trust and involvement of local leaders and communities, in their own language and in a context that empowers them not to comply with a central government or even a local physician or leader, but to own and promote the health service themselves. As the health promotion efforts progress, these potential pockets of late adopters need to be continuously reassessed and efforts modified to ensure that they are fully participating in the health services.

Throughout the history of disease eradication, examples can be drawn from several communication campaigns to exemplify this point. The successful efforts to eradicate smallpox are championed, primarily because they were successful rather than because they were well thought through or particularly persuasive: much of the smallpox effort was closer to coercion, particularly in the later stages. Coercion differs from persuasion in that persuasion leaves the final choice up to the individual or community in question. The failed attempt to eradicate malaria is often overlooked because it was ultimately unsuccessful; however there are good lessons to be learned from that period. Polio eradication stands out among eradication campaigns because it is a contemporary, high-profile, and well-documented effort that offers the public health

community a window into the internal dynamics of the communication elements behind successes and failures.

The Polio Experience

When the World Health Assembly passed the resolution to eradicate polio in
1988, it seemed a fairly feasible task. OPV was safe and easy enough to admin-
ister so that just about anyone could do it, provided that there was a functioning
cold chain and access to children. Countries and regions became increasingly
polio free, and it looked like the initiative was on track for the 2000 deadline.
As this deadline passed, the wild poliovirus was present in only a handful of
countries. Another year or so and transmission would easily be stopped, or so
it seemed (Figure 18.1).

As 2002 came, several countries faced great difficulty in reaching the necessary levels of population immunity. Polio continued to paralyze children
in high-rise communities in Cairo, hard to reach areas of Afghanistan and
Pakistan, and perhaps most strikingly in Nigeria, where high-profile resistance
to immunization in northern states was increasingly implicated in continued
transmission. In India, despite high levels of immunity in the majority of children across the country, the virus continued to circulate in the northern states
of Uttar Pradesh and Bihar, where populations were enduringly resistant to
immunization efforts. Important operational challenges existed, but the social
element was increasingly attributed to the failure to deliver OPV to vulnerable
children.

The initial reaction was to assume that ignorance or false beliefs constituted
the heart of resistance, which contradicted much of the contemporary development rhetoric. Research and cogent observation made it increasingly clear
that power relations based on social, cultural, economic, and political realities

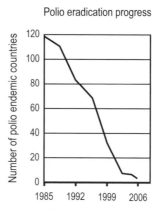

Figure 18.1   Progress in polio eradication (adapted from a presentation by Bruce R.
Aylward to the GPEI evaluation team in June 2009).

inspired opposition to the mass immunization efforts. Polio eradication planners began to respond to this reality in India in 2004, with the introduction of the "underserved strategy," which aimed to develop and nurture strategic partnerships and community ownership in areas resistant to polio campaigns. Local ownership lessened the resistance, which was ultimately not to the vaccine, but to the source from which it came—the central government—and the methods of delivery. These lessons continue to be applied to additional underserved groups in India, as the epidemiology of the polio virus has required the program to review continually its assessment of the underserved.

Although education and persuasion are, and will continue to be, important elements of any health campaign, the very local, sociopolitical sphere is often the level at which complex power relations and formations of social identity occur, requiring the most attention. This was accomplished in India and Nigeria. Drawing on these examples, let us examine how the polio eradication initiative has engaged late adopters at various levels of society.

Nigeria

Utilizing Traditional and Religious Leaders to Mobilize Resistant Communities for Polio Vaccination

Collaboration and partnership with traditional and religious leaders in Africa has long been an important strategy to successfully deliver health interventions to local populations. In Ghana and South Africa, local leaders have been instrumental in delivering messages about the dangers of HIV/AIDS since the early 1990s. In 1996, African leaders, both political and traditional, launched an enormous effort to improve the health of children across the continent and united to eradicate polio forever from the continent. Together the (then) Organization of African Unity pledged its determination to make Africa polio free.

In 2000, WHO, UNICEF and USAID jointly commissioned a study in Nigeria to examine priority communication channels for polio and routine immunization services. The study highlighted the importance of working with community leaders in rural and semirural areas of the country and confirmed the emerging practice of engaging traditional leaders to mobilize specific communities for the national immunization program (WHO, UNICEF and USAID 2000). Nonetheless, it took a national emergency and the near derailment of the global polio eradication initiative to reinforce the importance of working with traditional and religious leaders in Nigeria.

The Crisis

In 2003–2004, polio vaccination boycotts in Nigeria threatened global efforts to eradicate the disease. The ban by some northern states was brought about through unsubstantiated rumors that the vaccine was unsafe, could cause sterility, or spread HIV. Political motives were behind the circulation of these rumors, as some local leaders used the potential threat to the polio eradication program—a high-profile government initiative—as leverage to petition the central government for other demands. Once the rumors took hold, however, they became firmly entrenched in the community psyche and were implicated in wide-scale vaccine avoidance and subsequent boycott of polio campaigns in northern Nigeria. Entire villages of defiant communities were created; these groups were not laggards, they were hardcore resisters.

With public confidence shattered, the Nigerian government quickly mobilized traditional leaders to resolve the boycott and restore community support for the polio vaccine. After conflicting studies and reports were published on the safety of the polio vaccine, it was left to the Sultan of Sokoto, Alhaji Muhammadu Maccido, the spiritual head and spokesperson for the majority of Nigeria's Muslim population, to announce in early 2004 that the "oral polio vaccine is safe" (Renne 2006).

Rebuilding Trust

In September 2004, following the resumption of polio activities across the country, the Nigerian Federal Ministry of Health, with support from UNICEF and partners, organized a cross-border meeting of religious and traditional leaders in Kano. More than 150 sheiks, imams, mallams, and traditional leaders from Cameroon, Chad, Niger, Togo, Benin, and Burkina Faso joined together to share experiences and develop strategies in support of polio immunization. This served as an important first step in formalizing the roles and responsibilities of traditional leaders in the program. Traditional leader support was cemented in August 2005, when the Nigerian Forum of Religious and Traditional Leaders and the Media on Immunization and Child Survival was officially inaugurated by President Obasanjo (WHO 2011).

Polio eradication partners continued to work with traditional leaders through various initiatives, but the effort lacked national momentum and seemed consistently short of making a real impact. In February 2009, Bill Gates, on behalf of the Bill & Melinda Gates Foundation, which actively supports polio eradication efforts, visited Nigeria for the first time. During his visit he met national and state representatives as well as His Eminence, Sa'adu Abubakar, Sultan of Sokoto, to encourage his increasing involvement in the program. The Sultan obliged and soon addressed northern traditional leaders with a direct request for their heightened support for polio eradication. These leaders responded by inaugurating the Northern Traditional and Religious Leaders Forum for Primary Healthcare and Polio Eradication. This forum comprises emirs from twenty northern states, including the Federal Capital Territory, and has three primary objectives:

1. to improve immunization coverage and ensure interruption of wild poliovirus in Nigeria,
2. to support the strengthening of routine immunization in northern
   Nigeria, and
3. to contribute to the development of an effective primary health care
   system in northern Nigeria.

Although a number of technical and operational strategies as well as stronger
political ownership of the polio program by the Nigerian government at all levels have undoubtedly contributed to the significant reduction of Nigerian polio
cases in 2010, the systematic engagement of Nigeria's revered traditional leadership stands out as a pivotal contribution. It was instrumental in mobilizing
excluded populations who were critical for achieving universal immunization
coverage. Utilizing national and local leaders to reiterate consistent messages
on OPV safety helped reinstate public trust in immunization services, particularly in the North, while engendering local ownership and commitment to the
polio program.

In March 2010, the 19th Expert Review Committee (the national technical
advisory body responsible for oversight of polio eradication efforts in Nigeria)
specifically recognized the contributions traditional and religious leaders had
made to the country's sudden progress toward eradication, noting that the
"dramatic reduction of transmission of polioviruses" was achieved primarily
through improved coverage, which in turn was made possible through "the
deepening engagement of political and traditional leaders in polio eradication
in Nigeria." The 19th Expert Review Committee further expressed its belief
that "polio can be eradicated from Nigeria in 2010, if the commitment of political, government, and traditional leaders is sustained and strengthened..."
(Tomori et al. 2010).

In practice, traditional leaders in northern Nigeria have been engaged in
every Immunization Plus Day (IPD, or polio campaign) since October 2009.
Revered as royal fathers, several emirs have made strict public declarations
that polio eradication is a public health priority for all Nigerians (Figure 18.2).

District, village, and ward heads, who are representatives of the emirs, can
now be seen walking the dusty streets of northern Nigeria, working to ensure
polio teams reach every house in their community while also helping families
to understand, trust, and accept the vaccine by facilitating community dialogs
and public meetings. In the evenings, many traditional leaders attend the de-
briefing meetings at local health facilities, an activity they may have openly
resisted just a few years ago.

The Impact

This community engagement approach—coupled with improved operational
strategies to ensure that the vaccine is delivered to outlier communities—has

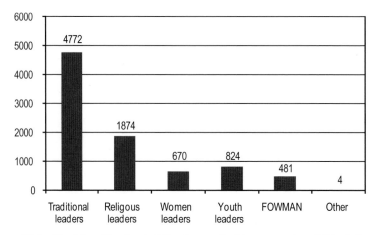

Figure 18.2 Traditional leaders in Nigeria now facilitate more than 60% of all community dialogs in northern Nigeria. Evidence from campaign monitoring indicates that more children are immunized in areas where traditional leaders lead efforts, such as dialogs (data from WHO campaign monitoring of IPDs, April 2010).

yielded considerable results in Nigeria. Since the committee's inauguration in August 2009, noncompliant households monitored throughout campaigns have fallen rapidly and, as a result, the levels of under-immunized children are dropping, particularly in northern states of Kano, Katsina, and Sokoto where the traditional system is strongest. As of November 2010, Nigeria has only eleven confirmed cases of wild poliovirus (six WPV1 and five WPV3) compared with 383 cases during the same period in 2009.

India

Engaging Migrant and Mobile Communities for Polio Vaccination in India

In 2002 and 2003, when the polio eradication program began to stumble in India, global partners needed a response. Polio cases in Muslim children were much higher than in the general population, and children in Muslim communities in northern India were not receiving OPV at the same rate as Hindu children. The resistance to immunization was volatile, and vaccinators, who were primarily Hindu, were not entirely accepted in Muslim communities.

Qualitative research in resistant areas revealed that resistance to immunization in primarily Muslim communities was not based on religious beliefs, as previously believed. Instead, it emerged from the sense of social identity, which was oppositional to the central government. Lack of trust in the government was borne out of years of marginalization and neglect, and thus was a logical response to the immunization services. In 2004, local influencers and religious leaders were brought into the program to convince resistant groups of underserved Muslim population that OPV was not a government strategy aimed at sterilizing their children and limiting population growth. Their help was crucial in bringing down resistance to OPV to record low levels in the program. However, this progress also revealed another group of underserved: migrants and mobile communities (WHO 2007b).

According to the 2001 census, the two polio endemic states of Uttar Pradesh and Bihar have the highest rates of out-migration in India. Approximately 5.13 million people move out of Uttar Pradesh annually, followed by Bihar which has 3.45 million people who travel largely in search of employment or better social opportunities. Between 2007 and 2009, 47% of the polio cases that occurred outside of the endemic states of Uttar Pradesh and Bihar were found to be multiple importations of wild poliovirus from either Central Bihar or Western Uttar Pradesh, according to Indian Ministry of Health monitoring data. The 17 polio type 1 cases reported in 2010 have almost all been detected in areas where the virus no longer circulates, and detailed epidemiological investigation undertaken by WHO's National Polio Surveillance Program has found 95% of these cases to be associated with mobile, migrant, or underserved populations.

Due to inadequate knowledge, insufficient demand, and disparate access to health services, migrant populations in Uttar Pradesh have been found to be almost twice as likely to have not been immunized with OPV as other population groups in the same area, according to monitoring data (Figure 18.3). A UNICEF-supported social survey undertaken in the highest-risk communities of Uttar Pradesh and Bihar found that only 51% of migrants and mobile communities in Uttar Pradesh knew where the polio vaccination booth was in their community, compared to the general population, where 95% knew where the booth was located during immunization campaigns (UNICEF 2010). With barriers to access and low demand, the probability that these mobile groups will receive every required dose of OPV rests almost entirely on whether or not they are identified, located, and engaged by mobile vaccination teams.

Based on their likelihood to miss doses of OPV and their role in maintaining and spreading polio transmission throughout India, mobile and migrant populations were added to the classification of "underserved" population groups in 2009.[1] With the trend of polio cases among Muslim populations reversed for the first time in 2008, and the epidemiology of the virus highlighting the vulnerability of mobile and migrant children, mobile and migrant groups were now characterized as the population most at risk for polio. Strategies to reach these groups with communication approaches and OPV vaccination now

---

[1]   The term underserved was coined in 2004 to describe efforts to improve immunization coverage in the primarily Muslim minority population group of northern India—the first group identified as disproportionately vulnerable to the polio virus.

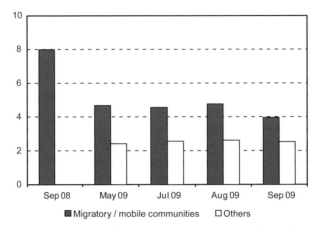

Figure 18.3 Migratory and mobile communities are almost twice as likely not to be immunized as the rest of the population, according to data presented by the National Polio Surveillance Project at the 21st India Expert Advisory Group for Polio Eradication meeting in November 2009.

comprise the "expanded underserved strategy," which has been embraced by the Indian Ministry of Health as the next strategic phase for polio eradication.

Avoiding Disparities in Migrants' Access to Health Services

Migrants in India have no entitlements to livelihood support systems or formal welfare schemes. Often they are not paid full wages because contractors deduct portions of their earnings as charge for securing employment. Migrants have limited bargaining power and greatly diminished social capital since they reside outside their familial or traditional social structures. With the additional burden posed by a lack of access to basic facilities, the results are borne mainly by women and children who suffer disproportionately in terms of disease burden and mortality. The vulnerability of nomadic groups is on par to that of migrants and is compounded further by their lack of legal residential status in many instances, their wariness of government-supported services, and the mutual reticence that health service providers and vaccinators feel about providing outreach services to these often clandestine groups.

It is therefore not surprising that migrants and nomadic groups are often left out of formal health services and lack the benefits offered through engagement with other social facilities such as education, clean water, and basic sanitation. In the Indian polio program, these populations represent the remaining groups yet to adopt healthy behaviors in general and OPV vaccination in particular. They comprise the weakest link that now challenges polio eradication in India.

To reach these groups with OPV vaccination, the polio eradication program first had to identify migrant groups, locate them, and employ an approach that reached every single child, as opposed to every single household. Subsequently, the program needed to develop appropriate ways to engage and involve these isolated groups in the eradication effort to ensure their full participation and ownership, similar to the way Muslim communities were engaged in the early days of the program.

Removing Impediments to Migrants' Access to Preventive and Curative Services

Utilizing experience from the underserved strategy to reach minority Muslims, the program immediately recognized that these groups had to be reached through trusted leaders and influencers from their own communities. In 2009, UNICEF's Social Mobilization Network (SMNet) identified and enlisted over 1300 nomadic informers in the seven highest risk districts of Uttar Pradesh. These mobilizers were chosen because they have social capital in these communities and can thus positively influence group behavior. Landlords, business owners, shopkeepers, and community leaders who are both well informed on population movements in and out of their district and influential and reliable in disseminating information were given preference in selection, and were sensitized regularly to the importance of reaching these groups with OPV vaccination. Each week they are contacted by a local SMNet worker to provide updates on incoming and outgoing population movements within their catchment area. Block mobilizers follow up on the leads, list all children under five years old, and turn the household list over to local officials and vaccination teams. As of September 2010, over 30,000 mobilizers in migrant communities had been identified in approximately 37,645 communities in Uttar Pradesh.

Once settlements are identified, a separate visit is undertaken to initiate discussion and disseminate messages on the importance of OPV and routine vaccination. Entrance into the community is facilitated by a trusted informant who has influence over the group. For most of these communities, literacy and knowledge is low, but OPV is largely accepted since it is the only public health service offered to them: "We take OPV because it is free of cost and Government is giving it to us at our doorstep"—nomadic mother in Western Uttar Pradesh (UNICEF 2010). Further evidence of this is found in a UNICEF 2009 communication review report on migrants and mobile communities in Badaun and Ghaziabad:

> Although uptake of polio immunization is fairly high among the target groups, there are key gaps in knowledge pertaining to immunization, polio itself, and other factors related to the disease. Indeed, when residents were asked about why they need to take repeated doses, many stated that this was the desire of the CMCs [community mobilization coordinators]; few were able to provide reasons for taking the OPV (Badaun).

> Making inroads in this area is facilitated by the fact that the communities, having traditionally been so excluded, welcome almost any service with openness given

the fact that they have been isolated from most basic services and amenities for
so long (Ghaziabad).

The identification of these communities was undertaken initially by SMNet
and vaccination teams, and access was facilitated by mobile vaccination teams,
which provided a critical entry point not only for increasing OPV vaccination
rates among these vulnerable groups, but also for the provision of wider health
services to help reduce vulnerability to poliovirus infection and other diseases.
Because vaccinators and social mobilization staff are essentially the only func-
tionaries who have reached out to these communities, migrants and nomadic
groups have begun to turn to these polio workers to fulfill their demands for a
wider range of other basic needs, including the provision of clean water, sanitation, and education.

Expanded messages on key healthy behaviors that could potentially inhibit poliovirus transmission are being introduced in these communities. Not
only do these additional interventions help to reduce polio risk factors (e.g.,
poor hygiene, sanitation, and nutritional status), they can also empower these
groups to take control of the health of their children and their families. The
extra services provided will additionally build goodwill, trust, and an enabling
environment for OPV vaccination.

Minimizing the Negative Impact of the Migration
Process on Health Outcomes

Population movement intensifies migrants' vulnerability to a wide range of
health risks, including polio, as migrants are more likely to miss out on OPV
doses than any other population group in India. The need to minimize the negative impact of the migration process on health outcomes, coupled with the
communication imperative to minimize the distance between the communication message and the provision of a service, has led to the adaptation of OPV
delivery system to reach Indian migrants as they travel.

For example, if you travel by train in Uttar Pradesh, Bihar, or Delhi during
a polio round, it would be difficult to miss the yellow polio banners draped
along stairwells, hung over platforms, and strung between arrival and depar-
ture announcement screens. Vaccinators clad in yellow vests work in each major entry point, searching for passing children under five years old to vaccinate.
This transit strategy has been in effect for over five years, with continuously
evolving innovations designed to reach and vaccinate the maximum number
of migrants in transit.

Communication channels have recently been expanded to maximize outreach to these groups while they travel, not only at train and bus stations, but
also through posters and hoardings at rest stops on major highways, through
visible booths placed along mela routes for traveling pilgrims to be vaccinated
as they make their religious treks, as well as on the border between Nepal

and India as migrants travel through the porous borders searching for work. Messaging has been more specifically targeted to migrants, highlighting the importance of getting vaccinated especially while traveling. Messages are disseminated on trains themselves, together with vaccination teams who travel on the most critical routes between Uttar Pradesh, Bihar, Delhi, and Maharashtra.

According to May 2010 monitoring data, 2,321,991 people in Uttar Pradesh and 1,898,494 in Bihar were vaccinated at train stations, melas, and bazaars.

Impact

It is premature to demonstrate the impact of the expanded underserved strategy; the intensified focus on these groups began less than one year ago and these groups continue to play a large role in persisting transmission in India. There is, however, evidence that the same strategy contributed to the significant reduction of cases among underserved Muslims since 2004, when the approach was first initiated (Figure 18.4). The Government of India and its partners are confident that the main principles of the underserved strategy—identifying and segmenting underserved groups, mobilizing credible local influencers to facilitate access and deliver messages, and utilizing communication messages and materials that are contextually relevant to segmented groups—are transferable to additional underserved communities. The Indian experience further demonstrates the need for communication programs that dynamically respond to continuous epidemiological assessments in an effort to identify underserved populations. Only then can universal coverage of all population groups be ensured at every stage of the program.

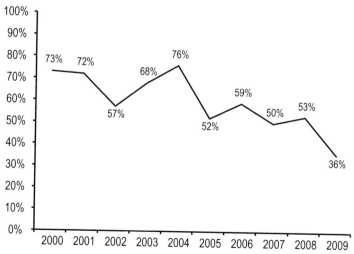

Figure 18.4   P1 cases among minority Muslims in Uttar Pradesh declined from 76% in 2004 to an all-time low of 35.7% in 2009.

Conclusion

Past eradication campaigns offer lessons to help us avoid repeating mistakes in future efforts. If applied, these lessons will also help the global public health community achieve better, timelier results for initiatives that aim to improve the general health and welfare of the world's growing population. Standard communication approaches have important contributions to make in support of any public health goal, but the nature of an eradication effort demands consideration and planning beyond the typical public health campaign. Our purpose in this chapter was to highlight areas where additional efforts and foresight are necessary, particularly in identifying and reaching out to marginalized groups in the early stages of the public health initiative.

Eradication efforts require both global advocacy and local communication that operate with a clear set of intended outcomes. Global efforts usually receive inspiration through a mandate from established bodies, such as the World Health Assembly, along with the coordinated efforts of a large donor and political community. The combined efforts of these bodies and institutions are critical for mobilizing the political and financial will necessary to persuade national governments to adopt public health interventions aimed at the eradication of a disease. A global communication strategy which inspires local campaigns to employ evidence-based, state-of-the-art approaches to health communication for behavior change is likely to succeed in moving a majority of the audience toward the end behavior, and thus closer to the eradication goal. It is important to recognize the important contribution that each of these elements can make toward the goal of eradication, as well as to identify the need to supplement large-scale approaches with local and more nuanced strategies.

In social and communication theory, it is accepted that people act on incentives and that the incentive for early and late majority adopters will be their health as well as the welfare of their loved ones. It is logical to assume that this powerful incentive is enough to move all people to adopt an end behavior. However, as we have illustrated here, the single incentive of personal welfare can be subverted by other incentives when some populations take oppositional positions to the public health good or fail to benefit from services offered. Thus, in addition to extending services into areas where people have traditionally been excluded, communication and incentives need to be highly localized and contextually adapted to motivate late adopters.

Fortunately, the polio eradication program and other public health activities offer successful examples of localized incentives. These include, but are not limited, to the following:

- Identify those populations likely to be left out of mass public health interventions during the beginning stages of the eradication effort; health and other social metrics are available and can be utilized to highlight where the eradication effort will likely confront challenges. It is not a

19

Group Report: Designing Elimination or Eradication Initiatives that Interface Effectively with Health Systems

Muhammad Ali Pate, John O. Gyapong,
Walter R. Dowdle, Adrian Hopkins, Dairiku Hozumi,
Mwelecele Malecela, and Stewart Tyson

Abstract

At the outset, disease eradication programs need to define short-, medium- and long-term goals and how these relate to and interact with the existing health system. Potential system synergies need to be evaluated on a country-by-country basis so that eradication efforts can be effectively integrated into existing government systems and processes. Critical to the success of any eradication program is the sense of "country ownership." Developing countries must be empowered and supported to take ownership and lead in the design and implementation of an eradication program. Consensus is necessary at the global level, but countries must have a voice in structuring eradication initiatives in their national contexts.

The global expectations that accompany a World Health Assembly (WHA) resolution must be understood by countries, particularly the need to strengthen health systems to achieve the goals inherent in an eradication program. Opportunities to bundle interventions should be explored and reporting mechanisms developed that derive from in-country reporting mechanisms. Objective metrics are needed along with explicit evaluations of health systems impacts. All programs should routinely undergo independent evaluation and corrective actions taken when necessary.

How Will the Health and Development Landscape Look over the Next 15 Years, and How Will This Influence Future Disease Eradication Programs?

Since the launch of the guinea worm and polio disease eradication programs in 1980 and 1988, respectively, the health and development landscape has changed dramatically. The architecture of global health aid has evolved into a complex entity involving the efforts of multiple donors and various stakeholders in an ever-increasing number of health initiatives. Low-income countries face many challenges: a double disease burden with the unfinished agenda of high levels of preventable and treatable infectious diseases is compounded by a mounting burden of noncommunicable diseases. Institutional capacity is often minimal and resources are limited. In the poorest countries, health systems are unable to deliver even the most basic services to its population. Overseeing and interacting with a large number of health partners and initiatives—some of whom work through parallel systems which may not be aligned with the country's national health plan nor reflected in a country's national budget—poses a formidable challenge to low-income countries (Schieber et al. 2006; Piva and Dodd 2009).

We expect that the global health situation will continue to evolve over the foreseeable future such that new disease eradication initiatives will operate in a very different environment than is currently in existence. Success of future disease eradication programs will depend on an understanding of how health systems are organized, financed, managed, and held accountable in low-income countries. In addition, we must be aware of the challenges that governments face when dealing with the increasingly complex development aid architecture and multiple aid delivery models. A multitude of parallel finance and delivery systems can easily overwhelm the already weak capacities in some countries (Hecht and Shah 2006).

Long-standing debates continue on the merits of targeted (vertical), health systems (horizontal), or combination (diagonal) approaches to improve health outcomes, and there is a growing appreciation of a combination (diagonal) approach, which optimizes the synergies between the two. Coexistence of future disease eradication programs and health systems-strengthening efforts will need to assure implementation of the most effective and efficient strategies to deliver maximum health gains, both in relation to eradication targets and in delivering a basic package of services that meet the health needs of the population (Mills 2005; Gyapong et al. 2010; Kabatereine et al. 2010). In our discussions, we explored a range of possible scenarios, based on the rapid pace of change since the WHA polio resolution in 1988. Broadly, we came to conclusions built around two possible scenarios.

The more optimistic scenario is that a growing global economy will create enabling opportunities for future disease eradication, subject to a robust investment case being made. There will be increasing global resources for health system development, with close alignment of national and global health interests through improved national coordination and leadership. Under this scenario, child mortality will continue to fall, and there will be no emerging pandemics. As the health of the population improves, global citizens will not tolerate continuing infectious diseases and will demand that governments eradicate specific diseases. Polio and guinea worm will be eradicated; however, polio will continue to incur ongoing costs in many countries due to national security concerns. Advances in technology will lead to price reductions of vaccines and other key commodities, enabling rapid expansion in the use of currently expensive vaccines and health-improving products.

The more pessimistic scenario is that there will be further fragmentation of the global health aid architecture, decreased health aid, and reduced effectiveness of much development assistance. Country capacities will be overwhelmed by many well-meaning but uncoordinated health initiatives that operate outside the national health plan and budget and incur high transaction costs. The minimal or absent health systems in the most challenged countries will lead donors to bypass struggling government systems and create parallel but unsustainable systems to deliver services. Government health budgets will increase slowly but will not keep pace with mounting disease burdens, due to both communicable and noncommunicable diseases. There will be increasing competition for health development assistance of new and old targeted health initiatives. Support for infectious diseases, immunization, or neglected tropical diseases (NTDs) will be squeezed by rising demands related to noncommunicable diseases, cancer, and health impacts from urbanization. New and uncertain agendas related to climate change will further constrain the fiscal space for health development. The tensions between national and globally defined health priorities will be exacerbated, leading some countries to reject disease eradication programs.

In either scenario, future disease eradication initiatives will need to present a robust investment case or business plan to address, at the very least, the following issues: the full estimated program costs; realistic time frames; potential impacts on the health system, both positive and negative (particularly impacts on human resources, finance, and service delivery); and clear ideas on how these impacts can be maximized or minimized. Disease eradication programs will also be required to optimize opportunities to deliver disease eradication packages in an integrated manner and to link with other priority programs and health system initiatives. They will need to define the criteria for success at different stages of the eradication pathway as well as the criteria for abandoning the goal of eradication. We anticipate that greater attention will be given to the strengthening of health systems. Imperative for the necessary agenda building are ongoing discussions between GAVI, GFATM, and the World Bank, the International Health Partnership Plus (IHP+), the US Global Health Initiative, and an increasing focus on results-based financing.

What Is the Optimal Interface (Best Fit) between Disease Eradication Programs and Health Systems?

Country health systems are heterogeneous in terms of their size, capacities, financing, structure, and ways of thinking about the world. There are different health system challenges in low- and middle-income countries and fragile states (Cavalli et al. 2010; Patel et al. 2010). Some countries with highly decentralized government systems face unique challenges (Oliveira Cruz and McPake 2010). Therefore, it is unlikely that one type of disease eradication program will fit all health systems. Thus, from the outset disease eradication programs will need to be flexible and adaptable to optimize how they interact with a particular health system context, within which they will operate and collaborate with health systems strengthening to find ways to work effectively to deliver short-, medium-, and long-term gains.

There is wide recognition that weak and failing health systems can undermine the success of an eradication program. Although disease eradication programs cannot be responsible to fix dysfunctional health systems, how they choose to operate can contribute to or undermine the long-term development of health systems.

Country ownership of disease eradication programs and health systems-strengthening initiatives are central to enabling lower-income countries to optimize the synergies between the two. The tensions between global partnerships and governments around issues of ownership and accountability need to be considered and openly addressed. An effective coordinating mechanism at the country level could play an important role in program success. Disease eradication programs should support the strengthening of government systems for planning and management, finance and accountability, monitoring, and evaluation. In the most challenging settings, this will need to be done in incremental steps. When government is in control, it is more likely that disease eradication programs will be "on plan and on budget," reflecting the priority within the national plan and national budget. Future disease eradication programs should seek to maximize the effectiveness of aid by providing resources through government finance channels, where these channels are robust. Where they are weak, the channels for providing resources will need to be addressed with other development partners.

Eventually, all disease eradication programs will end and the health system will need to absorb any ongoing long-term responsibilities. For example, after eradication, polio vaccines will need to be delivered through routine immunization systems for an undetermined time. Thus disease eradication programs need to build linkages and capacity with the health system early on in the program, with the end point and post-eradication periods in mind.

A major challenge is to balance the medium-term, results-driven disease eradication program agenda with the longer-term health system agenda to deliver comprehensive and sustainable services. The time frame of current disease eradication programs (e.g., in the case of polio, more than twenty years) highlights the importance of engaging closely with the health system from the planning phase.

Given the current fragmentation of the global health aid architecture, future disease eradication programs need to avoid developing "quick fix" parallel systems whenever possible. If parallel systems are absolutely necessary in the short term, plans must be in place to move rapidly to a medium- and longer-term model through engaging with a wider range of development partners.

Where a country's primary health care system is functioning well, disease eradication programs should use the existing system and hold governments accountable for results. Where a health system has broken down, disease eradication programs need to help rebuild it. There is evidence that fragile health systems are impacted disproportionately from global health initiatives. Positive synergies between disease-specific interventions and nontargeted health services are most likely to occur in robust health systems (Cavalli et al. 2010). Different models are needed according to the level of functionality of the primary health care system. The high transaction costs for disease eradication programs in under-resourced health systems can be reduced through greater integration or a bundling of services across multiple programs targeting the same populations.

The presence of private sector providers within country health systems is growing, both in the not-for-profit sector (e.g., faith-based health organizations) and the for-profit sector. The former group has collaborated with many disease eradication programs. While there has been less interaction with the private sector, for-profit organizations are increasingly playing important roles in providing preventive and curative health services, especially for urban and peri-urban populations in low- and middle-income countries. Because the government's regulatory oversight capacity is often inadequate, future disease eradication programs need to be aware of roles played by the for-profit providers and devise collaborative strategies to avoid creating pockets of unreached populations.

The following provide examples of good practice, where disease eradication programs have contributed to the strengthening of health services:

- The mass training of health workers (e.g., in conjunction with the polio initiative in India) demonstrates capacity building and demonstrates how an eradication program can strengthen the health system. However, the impact of all capacity-building efforts needs to be evaluated.
- Laboratory and surveillance systems developed in the polio eradication initiative can be transformed and used for broader infectious disease surveillance. In Nigeria, for example, polio laboratories can be used for measles and other disease surveillance.
- Procurement and logistics systems for disease eradication programs and vertical programs can be used for other health commodities, although experience in Senegal shows that this is difficult to achieve.
- Disease eradication programs provide an opportunity to integrate with other initiatives, such as expanded programs on immunization and vitamin A or the bundling of products in mass drug administrations. However, the integration of disease eradication programs with other

initiatives can also carry serious credibility risks, particularly if the promised additional items cannot be delivered in time or fall short in numbers.

Questions of the impact of targeted global health initiatives on efforts to strengthen national health systems led the WHO Positive Synergies Group and the IHP+ to establish indicators against each of the six core health system building blocks. The investment case for any future disease eradication program will need to delineate the potential interactions with each core system, including how the potential benefits could be maximized and the potential negative effects minimized or eliminated.

Do Current Disease Eradication Program Models Offer Lessons for the Design of Future Programs to Ensure an Effective Interface with Health Systems?

Formal health systems in developing countries often reach and stop at the district level. New models are needed to use existing community structures (e.g., as demonstrated by the African program for onchocerciasis control, polio, and guinea worm) in the context of health systems strengthening.

Disease eradication programs can increase financial and human resource flows at the community level and improve the effectiveness of the health system. Similarly, the evolution of global health initiatives in recent years offers lessons to the onchocerciasis, lymphatic filariasis, and polio eradication efforts in terms of how health systems can be strengthened (e.g., the GAVI, GFATM, World Bank common platform for health systems strengthening). A future disease eradication initiative must actively look at potential system synergies at the stage when they articulate the investment case.

Onchocerciasis

The history and development of the onchocerciasis program and the lessons that have been learned throughout are described by Hopkins (this volume). Here we wish to emphasize the remarkable advancement in efficiency and effectiveness that was achieved as the mass ivermectin treatment program evolved from reliance on unsustainable mobile teams to community-directed treatment. Communities became empowered to organize their own distribution in their own way at a time that suited the communities. Primary health care staff members at the periphery are now very much involved. Attitudes have changed from one of resistance, as they were often not included in the decision-making process, to one of full support, as they realize the usefulness of the community in the delivery of health care.

Sustainability plans for mass drug administration of ivermectin are now anchored at the health district level. Plans cover not only funding but also the roles of the various actors in the health district, including the community, and demonstrate health systems strengthening "from the bottom up."

As the vital link with the periphery, community ownership not only ensures implementation of the necessary high-coverage strategies to achieve elimination (Amazigo 2008), it remains the key to any changes in strategy that may be required to develop the elimination program. Community ownership and the associated strengthening of the health system has led to a whole series of health delivery strategies (called community-directed interventions) and will be central to efforts to control neglected tropical diseases, including the planned elimination of lymphatic filariasis.

Lymphatic Filariasis

The lymphatic filariasis model is based on the onchocerciasis model, which highlights the importance of mapping and baseline data from the very start, giving a much stronger base for monitoring. The model is more top-down than the onchocerciasis program and is tightly structured with time limits.

The Global Alliance to Eliminate Lymphatic Filariasis was established as the result of the World Health Assembly Resolution No. 52 of 1997, which targeted the elimination of lymphatic filariasis as a public health problem by the year 2020. All member states agreed to the resolution. The program employed mass drug administration of (a) Mectizan® and albendazole in Africa and (b) diethylcarbamizind in areas not endemic for onchocerciasis, based on research showing these to be effective microfilaricides capable of interrupting transmission when used for a period of not less than five years. The other mainstay of the program involves disease alleviation for those who already have the debilitating manifestations of the disease. This includes care of affected limbs through washing and elevation as well as surgery for those with hydroceles. To date, the program has delivered over 1 billion treatments in endemic countries. It has been described as the fastest growing program in public health (Molyneux 2009). However, although the program has been successful, some countries, particularly in Africa, have yet to start elimination programs (Gyapong and Twum-Danso 2006).

Mass drug administration has been implemented differently in the various countries but has remained a grassroots program. It involves villages, communes, and shehias where drugs are distributed house to house or at specific booths. The workforce used to distribute the drugs is named differently in the various countries, but it is basically comprised of community-based resource persons who are identified by the community to distribute the drugs. Studies in Nigeria, Cameroon, Ghana, Tanzania, and Kenya have shown (CDI Study Group 2010) that adding other responsibilities to the community health worker (i.e., distribution of nets) did not adversely affect delivery of ivermectin. To the contrary, this actually enhanced performance of the mass drug administration and any other interventions.

From a health systems perspective, efficient utilization of this workforce could and has, to a great extent, been shown to strengthen subdistrict-level health systems. The community workforce involved in mass drug administration offers an example of an effective framework to deliver interventions at the community level. In Tanzania, community volunteers (also referred to as "community own resource persons" or CORPs) have been able to act as support for patients following hydrocelectomy (Malecela et al. 2009), thus reducing the number of complications following surgery. CORPs have shown the ability to deliver several interventions such as long-lasting insecticide treated nets, vitamin A supplements, and mass drug administration, and this increased overall efficiency (WHO/TDR 2008). In Tanzania, the same CORPs are distributing drugs for five diseases as part of an integrated neglected tropical disease program (Malecela et al. 2009; Michael et al. 2008). The health system is broad, and this community health workforce is a crucial component, in particular for those systems that are already weak and fragmented. These examples clearly demonstrate where possibilities exist to find convergence with the health system.

Throughout the lymphatic filariasis program, there is strong country ownership. Countries decide how the program is implemented. Districts own their own aspects of the program and participate in the planning of the program. Data requirements are rigid, and national coordinating mechanisms are used to gather data. There are now moves to add anti-schistosomiasis and trachoma drugs, and use common systems for implementation.

Polio

Lessons learned throughout the polio eradication initiative have been summarized by Aylward (this volume) and are a valuable resource for any future eradication initiative. The global polio eradication initiative is anchored at the WHO in Geneva and has regional technical advisory groups (TAGs) and interagency coordination structures. At the country level, the program is built around the WHO expanded program on immunization, with replication of the regional TAG and interagency coordination committees at the national level. The strategy of the polio eradication initiative explicitly recognizes the importance of strengthening routine immunization and surveillance systems.

The polio eradication model has manifested synergy in areas such as its surveillance platform, which has been used for other infectious diseases (including measles, Japanese encephalitis, neonatal tetanus) as well as for early disaster warning systems (such as floods in Pakistan). However, results are mixed in the bundling of other interventions, such as bed nets and vitamin A.

The polio eradication initiative created a pilot program of results-based financing in Pakistan and Nigeria, through an innovative credit buy-down arrangement for polio vaccines. This allows partners, such as the Bill & Melinda Gates Foundation and Rotary International, to leverage their funds for purchasing vaccines and permit governments to receive the funds as in-kind grants, if results are achieved.

The polio eradication initiative could make a valuable contribution to the delineation of future disease eradication programs; however, additional independent evaluations are needed. We strongly recommend that documentation of the initiative be made available of the lessons that have been learned over the years.

What Are the Optimal Arrangements for Disease Eradication Programs in Relation to Health Systems Governance?

Key attributes of an optimal arrangement include issues related to governance, finance, management, and health human resources. To summarize our extensive discussions on the crucial elements necessary to achieve, when positioning a disease eradication program within the larger context of a health system, the components necessary to ensure optimal engagement are listed below.

1. Stewardship and Governance
    • Highest-level political commitment and ownership through a WHA resolution.
    • Informed by a robust evidence and investment case, based on broad consultation and consensus.
    • High-level technical leadership (usually WHO) with adequate capacity.
    • Active management following a WHA resolution, including building a wide national constituency for action.
    • An effective mechanism to engage global nongovernment partners (e.g., Rotary Club for polio, pharmaceutical industry for lymphatic filariasis).
    • Continued active reinforcement of national commitment to global eradication goals in the face of changes of governments.
    • Regional resolutions, committees, and TAGs important; regional operational forum can address cross-border issues; global and regional governance structures will need to be "light touch."
    • Clear, transparent mechanisms for flow of funds; role of ICCs at national and regional levels.
    • Optimize synergies across program and sectors, and with flexible and adaptable response in line with evolving global aid architecture.

- Need to examine what worked and did not work optimally in polio; mapping the governance structures involved in GPEI would be a useful exercise.

2. Planning and Management
   - Link global action plan to country priorities and national action plan.
   - Agreed realistic time frame at outset.
   - Establish criteria for exit point.
   - Map stakeholders, relations, and potential interactions with the health system.
   - Focus on management coordination and capacity development.

3. Service Delivery, Drugs, Commodities and Logistics
   - Improve access through functional infrastructure.
   - Align drug, vaccines, and commodities procurement and logistics systems where possible.
   - Integration of packages (e.g., mass drug administration) based on evidence within minimum service packages.

4. Finance
   - Resource mobilization for disease eradication programs should be additional so as not to distort ongoing programs at the global level (e.g., HIV vs. health systems).
   - Allocation decisions in-country should prioritize basic primary health services and support delivery of basic health care package.
   - Composition of spending should not undermine the functioning of health systems (e.g., salary bonuses, training workshops, per diems or large infrastructure without recurrent budget).
   - Structure financing in multi-year, predictable fashion and integrate within government budget cycle to ensure sustainability.
   - Include all local costs in national budget from the outset.
   - Improve government oversight on program spending to ensure efficiency and accountability.
   - Dedicated government counterpart contribution to support critical areas such as human resources.

5. Human Resources
   - Shift from single issue to multipurpose community-based workers.
   - Develop realistic incentive systems that do not compete with overall health system goals.
   - Plan transition strategy for workforce when end is in sight (e.g., how to redirect polio health workers in India).

6. Monitoring and Evaluation System
   - Maximize use of disease eradication program surveillance system and laboratory capacity for broader disease surveillance.
   - Link disease eradication program surveillance into national health information systems.

- Exact independent international technical evaluation of programs.
- Use common data systems where feasible.

Governance

The "optimal" governance arrangement for disease eradication programs will look differently from the perspective of disease eradication program funders or implementers at the various levels; that is, from global to country to local levels. Negotiating through the inherent tensions between global, regional, and national priorities as well as governance, finance, and human resources will be the key determinants of the success of future disease eradication programs (see also Stoever, this volume).

Governance and management of disease eradication programs must recognize the importance of government oversight, optimizing synergies, strengthening accountability, and the impact on country health systems. Within recipient countries, the Ministries of Health and disease eradication programs will need to jointly assess and determine which structures and systems must be strengthened to ensure implementation of the disease eradication program, so that parallel systems are not created specifically for the disease eradication program (see also Stoever et al., this volume). The disease eradication program should identify their investments in those systems. Ideally the systems strengthened will be ones that will remain after the disease eradication program has been completed. Given that fragile health systems suffer the most from global health initiatives, a sliding scale approach is needed when allocating disease eradication program and health systems-strengthening resources, so that the low-income countries receive the highest proportion of funding devoted to systems strengthening. Higher-income countries can then be allocated with less funding toward health systems strengthening.

Finance

Resource mobilization for a disease eradication program at the global level needs to be additional; that is, it should not displace funding intended for basic services and health systems. Further, the implication of dedicated disease eradication program funding at the national level needs to be considered. Countries should drive the resource allocation decision in their domains so that local priorities are not neglected in an attempt to support the global initiatives (Kirigia and Barry 2008).

The structure and composition of spending for global efforts need to be monitored to ensure that unnecessary distortions are not created. Governments need the flexibility to fill critical gaps related to implementation of the disease eradication program while simultaneously attending to other priorities (see also Jacobsen, this volume).

Funding large parallel initiatives through off-plan, off-budget mechanisms can make it very difficult for a country to predict its future resource expectations. Assuring stated commitments of governments to eradication programs may require additional counterpart funding dedicated to critical areas such as the health workforce.

Management

All global health initiatives, including eradication programs, need to be aligned with and embedded within national health plans so that they reflect country priorities. Disease eradication programs need to pursue specific goals and contribute to wider efforts to strengthen health systems (see also Tyson and Biellik, this volume).

Where regular health information systems may not satisfy the requirements of a disease eradication program, adjustments in reporting arrangements may have to be made. If parallel systems have to be created in the short term, inter-operability of the data systems and linkages need to be secured (see also Hinman, this volume).

Health Human Resources

By definition, disease eradication programs require extra effort in addition to ongoing routine work, which may mean hiring temporary workers to operate at the community level. Even when these workers are volunteers, there is often the need to remunerate as well as manage and supervise this group of community workers. The disease eradication program may need to mobilize and provide for the additional funds in consultation with the Ministries of Health (Rowden 2010).

To strengthen the workforce within the health system, the ideal community worker will be multi-skilled rather than a "single-disease" worker (see also Bates et al., this volume). This implies the need for adequate training curricula, materials, and resources (Vujicic 2010; Fulton et al. 2011).

Salary benefits and differential rates across different initiatives distort the management of the health system and can be counterproductive unless managed carefully (see also Hanvoravongchai et al., this volume). When incentives need to be provided, monetary as well as nonmonetary incentives should be considered. Professional performance bonuses granted as lump sum amounts to subdistrict-level workers were, for example, found to be acceptable in Tanzania. In the Congo, however, when graduated lump sums were allocated to the health workforce, the outcome was highly inequitable.

Over the course of implementing a disease eradication program, a transition strategy must be developed to secure the engaged workforce after the completion of a disease eradication program. For example, in the case of the polio program in India, which currently engages more than half a million health workers, what happens after the program is over has serious implications for those involved. Without a good transition strategy, the possibility of negative incentives developing among the workers cannot be excluded.

Recommendations

In addressing the question of how a future eradication program can be designed to interface most effectively with the health system in which it is operating, we offer the following recommendations:

1. Disease eradication programs should evaluate potential system syner- gies in each country with the goal of strengthening and integrating with existing government systems and processes wherever feasible. Disease eradication programs should be flexible to adapt to country situations without losing focus of their primary objective.

2. Developing countries should be empowered and aided to own and lead the design and implementation of the disease eradication programs in their own contexts. While consensus is reached at the global level, countries must have a say as to how the initiatives are structured in their own contexts. Country ownership is a critical factor for success.

3. Disease eradication programs should be adapted to each country's cir- cumstances. There is no "one size fits all" approach. A sliding scale ap- proach should be implemented, where the most fragile health systems are allocated more resources for health systems strengthening.

4. Countries should understand global expectations, and vice versa, when supporting a WHA resolution on disease eradication, particularly in re- gard to the need to strengthen health systems to achieve disease eradi- cation program goals.

5. Disease eradication programs should explore opportunities to deliver disease eradication packages in an integrated manner and bundle in- terventions without losing focus of their own objectives and interven- tions, as with mass drug administration for NTDs.

6. Reporting mechanisms used in eradication programs should be devel- oped and derived from in-country reporting mechanisms (e.g., the case of the Ghana SWAp). In doing so, the decentralization context should be taken into account.

7. Disease eradication programs should develop objective metrics and include explicit evaluations of health systems impacts. All programs should be independently evaluated for lessons learned and corrective actions taken when necessary.

8. From the outset, disease eradication programs should define short-, me- dium-, and long-term goals and their relationship to the health system. For example, when building laboratory capacity, a short-term focus

could be human resource technical assistance and training. On the medium term, this could include logistics support and equipment, whereas on the longer term, this may consist of infrastructure development such as improved laboratories for wider use in other diseases, institutionalizing human resources, and funding into government budget.

List of Acronyms

ACSD	Accelerated Child Survival and Development program
AIDS	acquired immunodeficiency syndrome
AMEAs	accelerated measles elimination activities
ANC	antenatal care
APOC	African Program for Onchocerciasis Control
BCA	benefit-cost analysis
BCG	Bacille Calmette-Guérin
BMGF	Bill & Melinda Gates Foundation
CDC	Centers for Disease Control and Prevention
CDI	community-directed intervention
CDTI	community-directed treatment with ivermectin
CEA	cost-effectiveness analysis
CORPs	community own resource persons
CRS	congenital rubella syndrome
DALY	disability-adjusted life years
DEC	diethylcarbamazine
DFID	Department for International Development
DTP	diphtheria, pertussis, tetanus
EIC	eradication investment case
EIR	entomological inoculation rate
EPI	expanded program on immunization
GAO	Government Accountability Office
GAVI	Global Alliance for Vaccines and Immunization
GDP	gross domestic product
GFATM	Global Fund to fight AIDS, Tuberculosis, and Malaria
GHIs	global health initiatives
GHWA	Global Health Workforce Alliance
GNI	gross national income
GPEI	Global Polio Eradication Initiative
GPG	global public good
HAT	human African trypanosomiasis
Hib	*Haemophilus influenzae* type b
HIV	human immunodeficiency virus
HPV	human papilloma virus
ICC	interagency coordination committee
ICER	incremental cost-effectiveness ratio
ICT	immunochromatography
IFFIm	International Finance Facility for Immunization
IHP+	International Health Partnership Plus

IMCI	Integrated Management of Childhood Illnesses
IMF	International Monetary Fund
INB	incremental net benefits
IPD	immunization plus day
IPTp	intermittent preventive treatment in pregnancy
ITFDE	International Task Force for Disease Eradication
ITI	International Trachoma Initiative
ITN	insecticide-treated nets
JE	Japanese encephalitis
JLI	Joint Learning Initiative
LAC	Latin America and Caribbean countries
LF	lymphatic filariasis
LSHTM	London School of Hygiene & Tropical Medicine
MalERA	malaria eradication research agenda
MCH team	mother and child health team
MCV	measles-containing vaccine
MDA	mass drug administration
MMR	measles-mumps-rubella
MR	measles-rubella
NGDO	nongovernmental development organization
NGO	nongovernmental organization
NIAID	National Institute of Allergy and Infectious Diseases
NNT	neonatal tetanus
NTD	neglected tropical disease
OCP	Onchocerciasis Control Program
OECD	Organisation for Economic Co-operation and Development
OEPA	Onchocerciasis Elimination Program for the Americas
OPV	oral poliovirus vaccine
PAHO	Pan American Health Organization
PATTEC	Pan African Tsetse and Trypanosomiasis Eradication Campaign
PCR	polymerase chain reaction
PCT	preventive chemotherapy
PPP	purchasing power parity
QALY	quality-adjusted life years
REMO mapping	rapid epidemiological mapping of onchocerciasis
R-PRGs	Regional Program Review Groups
SAE	severe adverse experience
SAFE strategy	surgery, antibiotics, face washing, and environmental improvement
SARS	severe acute respiratory syndrome
SIA	supplementary immunization activity
SMNet	social mobilization network

STAG	Strategic and Technical Advisory Group
STDs	sexually transmitted diseases
SWOT	strengths, weaknesses, opportunities and threats
TAG	Technical Advisory Group
TB	tuberculosis
TDR	Special Programme for Research & Training in Tropical Diseases
TT	tetanus toxoid vaccine
UNICEF	United Nations Children's Fund
USAID	U.S. Agency for International Development
WHA	World Health Assembly
WHO	World Health Organization
WPV	wild poliovirus

Bibliography

Note: Numbers in square brackets denote the chapter in which an entry is cited.

Ahmad, K. 2003. Tsetse eradication programme under fire. *Lancet Infect. Dis.* **3(1)**:4. [6]

Ahorlu, C., S. Dunyo, E. Afrai, K. Koram, and F. Nkrumah. 1997. Malaria-related beliefs and behaviour in southern Ghana: Implications for treatment, prevention and control. *Trop. Med. Intl. Health* **2(5)**:488–499. [12]

Alexander, L. N., J. F. Seward, T. A. Santibanez, et al. 2004. Vaccine policy changes and epidemiology of poliomyelitis in the United States. *JAMA* **292(14)**:1696–1701. [9]

Amazigo, U. V. 2008. The African Programme for Onchocerciasis Control (APOC). *Ann. Trop. Med. Parasitol.* **102(1)**:19–22. [19]

Anderson, R. M., and R. May. 1991. Infectious Diseases of Humans: Dynamics and Control. Oxford: Oxford Univ. Press. [5]

Andreasen, A., and P. Kotler. 2008. Strategic Marketing for Nonprofit Organizations, 7th ed. Saddle River, NJ: Pearson Education, Inc. [12]

Andrews, J. M., and A. D. Langmuir. 1963. The philosophy of disease eradication. *Am. J. Public Health* **53**:1–6. [1]

Andrus, J. K., C. A. de Quadros, and C. Castillo-Solórzano. 2011a. Chapter 54: Measles. In: Tropical Infectious Diseases: Principles, Pathogens and Practice, ed. R. L. Guerrant et al. New York: Saunders, in press. [3]

Andrus, J. K., C. A. de Quadros, C. Castillo-Solórzano, M. Roses Periago, and D. A. Henderson. 2011b. Measles and rubella eradication in the Americas. *Vaccine*: in press. [3]

Andrus, J. K., C. A. de Quadros, C. Ruiz Matus, S. Luciani, and P. Hotez. 2009. New vaccines for developing countries: Will it be feast or famine? *Am. J. Law Medicine* **35**:311–322. [3]

Andrus, J. K., V. Dietz, J. W. Fitzsimmons, and C. Castillo-Solórzano. 2006. Accelerating policy, deployment, and access to new and underutilized vaccines in developing countries. *Harvard Health Policy Rev.* **7(2)**:91–101. [3]

Andrus, J. K., A. M. Ropero, G. Ghisays, et al. 2010. Yellow fever and health diplomacy. In: Negotiating and Navigating Global Health: Case Studies in Global Health Diplomacy, ed. E. Rosskam and I. Kickbusch. London: World Scientific, Imperial College Press. [3]

Andrus, J. K., and M. Roses Periago. 2004. Elimination of rubella and congenital rubella syndrome in the Americas: Another opportunity to address inequities in health. *Pan. Am. J. Public Health* **15**:145–146. [3]

APOC. 2009. Community directed treatment with ivermectin (CDTI). www.who.int/apoc/cdti/en (accessed 17 February 2011). [4]

Arora, N. K., S. Chaturvedi, and R. Dasgupta. 2010. Global lessons from India's poliomyelitis elimination campaign. *Bull. WHO* **88(3)**:161–240. [16]

Arora, N. K., A. K. Patwari, and M. Lakshman, eds. 1999. Pulse Polio Immunization Program Evaluation 1997–1998. New Delhi: All India Institute of Medical Sciences. [16]

Atun, R., S. Bennett, and A. Duran. 2008. When do vertical (stand-alone) programmes have a place in health systems? Policy brief written for the WHO European Ministerial Conference on Health Systems, June 25–27, 2008, Tallinn, Estonia. http://www.euro.who.int/__data/assets/pdf_file/0008/75491/E93417.pdf (accessed 11 October 2010). [1]

Atun, R., T. de Jongh, F. Secci, K. Ohiri, and O. Adeyi. 2010. Integration of targeted health interventions into health systems: A conceptual framework for analysis. *Health Policy Plan.* **25**:104–111. [15, 17]

Atun, R., N. Lennox-Chhugani, F. Drobniewski, Y. A. Samyshkin, and R. J. Coker. 2004. A framework and toolkit for capturing the communicable disease programmes within health systems: Tuberculosis control as an illustrative example. *Eur. J. Public Health* **14(3)**:267–273. [17]

Auld, M. C. 2003. Choices, beliefs, and infectious disease dynamics. *J. Health Econ.* **22(3)**:361–377. [5]

Aylward, R. B., A. Acharya, S. England, M. Agocs, and J. Linkins. 2003. Global health goals: Lessons from the worldwide effort to eradicate poliomyelitis. *Lancet* **362(9387)**:909–914. [2, 9, 16]

Aylward, R. B., K. A. Hennessey, N. Zagaria, J. M. Olivé, and S. L. Cochi. 2000a. When is a disease eradicable? 100 years of lessons learned. *Am. J. Public Health* **90**:1515–1520. [1, 5, 7, 8, 16]

Aylward, R. B., H. F. Hull, S. L. Cochi, et al. 2000b. Disease eradication as a public health strategy: A case study of poliomyelitis eradication. *Bull. WHO* **78**:285–297. [1]

Aylward, R. B., and J. Linkins. 2005. Polio eradication: Mobilizing and managing the human resources. *Bull. WHO* **83(4)**:268–273. [2, 16, 17]

Aylward, R. B., R. W. Sutter, S. L. Cochi, et al. 2006. Risk management in a polio-free world. *Risk Analysis* **26**:1441–1448. [2]

Barrett, S. 2003. Global disease eradication. *J. Eur. Econ. Assoc.* **1(2/3)**:591–600. [9]

———. 2004. Eradication versus control: The economics of global infectious disease policies. *Bull. WHO* **82**:683–688. [1, 5, 8, 9]

———. 2006. The smallpox eradication game. *Public Choice* **130(1–2)**:179–207. [5, 9]

———. 2007. Why Cooperate? The Incentive to Supply Global Public Goods. Oxford: Oxford Univ. Press. [8]

———. 2009. Polio eradication: Strengthening the weakest links. *Health Affairs* **28(4)**:1079–1090. [5]

Barrett, S., and M. Hoel. 2003. Optimal Disease Eradication. Oslo: Health Economics Research Programme, Univ. of Oslo. [5]

———. 2007. Optimal disease eradication. *Env. Dev. Econ.* **12**:627–652. [5, 9]

Bauch, C. T., and D. J. D. Earn. 2004. Vaccination and the theory of games. *PNAS* **101(36)**:13,391–13,394. [5]

Bauch, C. T., A. P. Galvani, and D. J. D. Earn. 2003. Group interest versus self-interest in smallpox vaccination policy. *PNAS* **100(18)**:10,564–10,567. [5]

Beauchamp, D. E. 2007. Community: The neglected tradition of public health. In: Public Health Ethics: Theory, Policy, and Practice, ed. R. Bayer et al., pp. 45–56. Oxford: Oxford Univ. Press. [11]

Béhague, D. P., and K. T. Storeng. 2008. Collapsing the vertical-horizontal divide: An ethnographic study of evidence-based policymaking in maternal health. *Am. J. Public Health* **98(4)**:644–649. [15]

Beutels, P., W. J. Edmunds, and R. D. Smith. 2008. Partially wrong? Partial equilibrium and the economic analysis of public health emergencies of international concern. *Health Econ.* **17(11)**:1317–1322. [9]

Bhattacharya, S., and R. Dasgupta. 2009. A tale of two global health programs: Smallpox eradication's lessons for the antipolio campaign in India. *Am. J. Public Health* **99(7)**:1176–1184. [5]

Bhutta, Z. A., S. Ali, S. Cousens, et al. 2008. Alma-Ata: Rebirth and Revision 6. Interventions to address maternal, newborn, and child survival: What difference can integrated primary health care strategies make? *Lancet* **372**:972–989. [15]

Black, R. E., S. S. Morris, and J. Bryce. 2003. Where and why are 10 million children dying every year? *Lancet* **361**:2226–2234. [15]

Blacklock, D. B. 1926. The development of *Onchocerca volvulus* in *Simulium damnosum*. *Ann. Trop. Med. Parasitol.* **20**:1–48. [4]

Blenko, M., M. Mankins, and P. Rogers. 2010. The decision-driven organization. *Harvard Bus. Rev.* **88(6)**:54–62. [12]

Bloch, A. B., W. A. Orenstein, H. C. Stetler, et al. 1985. Health impact of measles vaccination in the United States. *Pediatrics* **76**:524–532. [3]

Bloom, D. E. 2007. Governing global health. *Finance & Devel.* **44**:31–35. [16]

Boatin, B. 2008. The onchocerciasis control program in West Africa (OCP). *Ann. Trop. Med. Parasitol.* **102(1)**:1317. [4]

Braber, K. L. 2004. An evaluation of GAEL, the Global Alliance for the Elimination of Leprosy. *Leprosy Rev.* **75**:208–213. [13]

Bradley, D. J. 1998. The particular and the general: Issues of specificity and verticality in the history of malaria control. *Parassitologia* **40(1–2)**:5–10. [17]

Brandach, J. 1996. Organizational Alignment: The 7-S Model. Boston: Harvard Business School Publishing. [12]

Brisson, M., and W. J. Edmunds. 2003. Economic evaluation of vaccination programs: The impact of herd-immunity. *Med. Decis. Making* **23(1)**:76–82. [9]

Broekmans, J. F., G. B. Migliori, and H. L. Rieder. 2002. European framework for tuberculosis control and elimination in countries with a low incidence: Recommendations of the World Health Organization (WHO), International Union Against Tuberculosis and Lung Disease (IUATLD) and Royal Netherlands Tuberculosis Association (KNCV) Working Group. *Eur. Respir. J.* **19**:765–775. [6]

Bryce, J., K. Gilroy, G. Jones, et al. 2010. The Accelerated Child Survival and Development programme in west Africa: A retrospective evaluation. *Lancet* **375**:572–582. [15]

Buse, K., and A. M. Harmer. 2007. Seven habits of highly effective global public-private health partnerships: Practice and potential. *Soc. Sci. Med.* **64(2)**:259–271. [16]

Bush, K. 2000. Polio, war and peace. *Bull. WHO* **78**:281–282. [2]

Cairncross, S., F. Cutts, and H. Periés. 1997. Dracunculiasis eradication. *Lancet* **350(9080)**:812–813. [17]

Caplan, A. 2009. Is disease eradication ethical? *Lancet* **373**:2192. [8]

Carter Center. 2010. International Task Force. http://www.cartercenter.org/health/itfde/index.html (accessed 23 October 2010). [1]

Cassels, A. 1997. A Guide to Sector-wide Approaches for Health Development: Concepts, Issues and Working Arrangements. Geneva: WHO. [16]

Castillo-Solórzano, C., and J. K. Andrus. 2004. Rubella elimination and improving health care for women. *Emerg. Infect. Dis.* **10**:2017–2021. [3]

Castillo-Solórzano, C., and C. A. de Quadros. 2002. Accelerated rubella control and the prevention of congenital rubella syndrome. *Pan Am. J. Public Health* **11(4)**:273–276. [3]

Castillo-Solórzano, C., C. Marsigli, P. Bravo Alcantara, et al. 2008. Progress toward elimination of rubella and congenital rubella syndrome: The Americas, 2003–2008. *MMWR* **57(43)**:1176–1179. [3]

Cavalli, A., S. I. Bamba, M. N. Traore, et al. 2010. Interactions between global health initiatives and country health systems: The case of a neglected tropical diseases control program in Mali. *PLoS Negl. Trop. Dis.* **4(8)**:e798. [15, 19]

CDC. 1993a. Initial therapy for tuberculosis in the era of multidrug resistance: Recommendations of the Advisory Council for the Elimination of Tuberculosis. *MMWR* **42(RR–7)**:1. [6]

———. 1993b. Recommendations of the International Task Force for disease eradication. *MMWR* **42(RR-16)**:1–38. [6, 7]

———. 1996. Progress toward the elimination of neonatal tetanus: Egypt, 1988–1994. *MMWR* **45(04)**:89–92. [6]

———. 1998. Progress toward the elimination of tuberculosis: United States, 1998. *MMWR* **48(33)**:732–736. [6]

———. 1999a. Global disease elimination and eradication as public health strategies. *MMWR* **48(Suppl)**:1–211. [1]

———. 1999b. The principles of disease elimination and eradication. *MMWR* **48(Suppl 1)**:23–27. [3]

CDI Study Group. 2010. Community-directed interventions for priority health problems in Africa: Results of a multicountry study. *Bull. WHO* **88(7)**:509–518. [19]

Cello, J., A. V. Paul, and E. Wimmer. 2002. Chemical dynthesis of poliovirus cDNA: Generation of infectious virus in the absence of natural template. *Science* **297**:1016–1018. [1, 5]

Chan, M. 2008. The Case for Completing Polio Eradication. Geneva: WHO Report. [8]

———. 2010. Time to get back on track to meet the millennium development goals. Opening address, Director-General of WHO. http://www.who.int/dg/speeches/2010/WHA_address_20100517/en/index.html (accessed 21 October 2010). [15]

Chen, L. C., and G. Berlinguer. 2001. Health equity in a globalizing world. In: Challenging Inequities in Health: From Ethics to Action, ed. T. Evans. Oxford: Oxford Univ. Press. [8]

Chu, B. K., P. J. Hooper, M. Bradley, D. A. McFarland, and E. A. Ottesen. 2010. The economic benefits resulting from the first 8 years of the global programme to eliminate lymphatic filariasis (2000–2007). *PLoS Negl. Trop. Dis.* **4(6)**:e708. [6, 13]

Cialdini, R. 2001. Harnessing the science of persuasion. *Harvard Bus. Rev.* **October**:72–79. [12]

Clements, C. J., and F. T. Cutts. 1995. The epidemiology of measles: Thirty years of vaccination. *Curr. Topics Microbiol.* **191**:13–33. [3]

Cochi, S. L., C. A. de Quadros, S. Dittman, et al. 1998. What are the societal and political criteria for eradication? In: The Eradication of Infectious Diseases, ed. W. R. Dowdle and D. R. Hopkins, pp. 157–175. Dahlem Workshop Report, J. Lupp, series ed. Chichester: John Wiley & Sons. [1, 2, 7]

Coles, J. 2006. Blindness and the Visionary: The Life and Work of Sir John Wilson. London: Giles de la Mar Publishing. [4]

Collins, J. 2001. Level 5 Leadership. *Harvard Bus. Rev.* **January**:67–76. [12]

Creese, A. L., and R. H. Henderson. 1980. Cost-benefit analysis and immunization programmes in developing countries. *Bull. WHO* **58(3)**:491–497. [9]

Crisp, G. 1956. Simuluium and Onchocerciasis in the Northern Territories of the Gold Coast. London: British Empire Society for the Blind. [4]

Cummings, T., and C. Worley. 1996. Organizational Development and Change, p. 467. Boston: Southwestern College Publishing. [12]

Cutting, W. A. M. 1980. Cost-benefit evaluations of vaccination programmes. *Lancet* **2(8195)**:634–636. [9]

Cutts, F. T., and L. E. Markowitz. 1994. Successes and failures in measles control. *J. Infect. Dis.* **170(Suppl 1)**:S32–S41. [3]

Dabbagh, A., M. Gacic-Dobo, and E. Simons. 2009. Global measles mortality, 2000–2008. *MMWR* **58(47)**:1321–1326. [17]

Dadzie, Y., M. Neira, and D. Hopkins. 2003. Final report of the conference on the eradicability of onchocerciasis. *Filaria J.* **2**:2. [4]

Danovaro-Holiday, M. C., A. M. Ropero, and J. K. Andrus. 2008. Progress in vaccination against *Hemophilus influenzae* type b in the Americas. *PLoS Med.* **5(4)**:e87. [3]

Dawson, A. 2009. Transparency, accountability and vaccination policy. *J. Med. Ethics* **35(5)**:274. [8]

Dentzer, S. 2008. Past, present and future partnerships in disease elimination and eradication. The Carter Center. http://www.gsk.com/community/filariasis/downloads/Partnerships-in-disease-elimination-Report.pdf (accessed 23 October 2010). [13]

de Quadros, C. A., J. K. Andrus, M. C. Danovaro-Holliday, and C. Castillo-Solórzano. 2008. Feasibility of global measles eradication after interruption of transmission in the Americas. *Expert Rev. Vaccines* **7(3)**:355–362. [3, 17]

de Quadros, C. A., J. M. Olive, B. S. Hersh, et al. 1996. Measles elimination in the Americas: Evolving strategies. *JAMA* **13**:224–229. [3]

DeRoeck, D. 2004. The importance of engaging policy-makers at the outset to guide research on and introduction of vaccines: The use of policy-maker surveys. *J. Health Popul. Nutr.* **22(3)**:322–330. [7]

De Serres, G., N. J. Gay, and C. P. Farrington. 2000. Epidemiology of transmissible diseases after elimination. *Am. J. Epidemiol.* **151**:1039–1048. [1]

DFID. 2007. The international health partnership. http://webarchive.nationalarchives.gov.uk/+/http://www.dfid.gov.uk/Media-Room/News-Stories/2007/The-International-Health-Partnership-Launched-Today/ (accessed 1 December 2010). [16]

Dias, J. C. 2007. Southern Cone Initiative for the elimination of domestic populations of *Triatoma infestans* and the interruption of transfusional Chagas disease. Historical aspects, present situation, and perspectives. *Memórias do Instituto Oswaldo Cruz* **102(Suppl. 1)**:11–8. [6]

———. 2009. Elimination of Chagas disease transmission: Perspectives. *Memórias do Instituto Oswaldo Cruz* **104**:41–45. [6]

Diawara, L., M. O. Traoré, A. Badji, et al. 2009. Feasibility of onchocerciasis elimination with ivermectin treatment in endemic foci in Africa: First evidence from studies in Mali and Senegal. *PLoS Negl. Trop. Dis.* **3(7)**:e497. [4]

Dobson, M. 2007. Disease: The Extraordinary Stories Behind History's Deadliest Killers. London: Quercus Publishing Plc. [8]

Donnelly, M. J., B. C. Herold, S. G. Jenkins, and R. S. Daum. 2003. Obstacles to the elimination of *Haemophilus influenzae* type b disease: Three illustrative cases. *Pediatrics* **112(6)**:1465–1466. [6]

Dowdle, W. R. 1998. The principles of disease elimination and eradication. *Bull. WHO* **76(2)**:22–25. [1, 5, 8]

Dowdle, W. R., and D. R. Hopkins, eds. 1998. The Eradication of Infectious Diseases. Dahlem Workshop Report, J. Lupp, series ed. Chichester: John Wiley & Sons. [1, 2, 7, 16]

Drucker, P. 2001. The Essential Drucker. New York: HarperCollins. [12]

Duintjer Tebbens, R. J., M. A. Pallansch, S. L. Cochi, et al. 2011. Economic analysis of the global polio eradication initiative. *Vaccine* **29**:334–343. [1, 5, 8–11]

Duintjer Tebbens, R. J., M. A. Pallansch, O. M. Kew, et al. 2006a. Risks of paralytic disease due to wild or vaccine-derived poliovirus after eradication. *Risk Analysis* **26(6)**:1471–1505. [9]

———. 2005. A dynamic model of poliomyelitis outbreaks: Learning from the past to help inform the future. *Am. J. Epidemiol.* **162(4)**:358–372. [9]

———. 2008. Uncertainty and sensitivity analyses of a decision analytic model for post-eradication polio risk management. *Risk Analysis* **28(4)**:855–876. [9]

Duintjer Tebbens, R. J., N. Sangrujee, and K. M. Thompson. 2006b. The costs of polio risk management policies after eradication. *Risk Analysis* **26(6)**:1507–1531. [9]

Duintjer Tebbens, R. J., and K. M. Thompson. 2009. Priority shifting and the dynamics of managing eradicable infectious diseases. *Manag. Sci.* **55(4)**:650–663. [9, 10]

Duke, B. O. L., and J. Anderson. 1972. A comparaison of the lesions produced in the corna of the rabbit eye by microfilaria of the forest and Sudan-Savannah strains of *Onchocerca volvulus* from Cameroon. *Tropenmed. Parasitol.* **23**:354–368. [4]

Duke, B. O. L., and A. Garner. 1976. Fundus lesions in the rabbit eye following inoculation of *Onchocerca volvulus* in the posterior segment. *Tropenmed. Parasitol.* **27**:3–17. [4]

Dye, C., and B. G. Williams. 2008. Eliminating human tuberculosis in the twenty-first century. *J. R. Soc. Interface* **5(23)**:653–662. [6]

Edmunds, W. J., G. F. Medley, and D. J. Nokes. 1999. Evaluating the cost-effectiveness of vaccination programmes: A dynamic perspective. *Stat. Med.* **18(23)**:3263–3282. [9]

Eisenhardt, K., J. Kahwajy, and L. J. Bourgeois, III. 1997. How Teams Have a Good Fight. Boston: Harvard Business Review. [12]

Ekman, G., I. Pathmanathan, and J. Liljestrand. 2008. Alma-Ata: Rebirth and Revision 7. Integrating health interventions for women, newborn babies, and children: A framework for action. *Lancet* **372**:990–1000. [15]

El-Sayed, N., Y. El-Gamel, A. A. Abbassy, et al. 2008. Monovalent type 1 oral poliovirus vaccine in newborns. *N. Engl. J. Med.* **359(16)**:1655–1665. [2]

Emerson, C., and P. Singer. 2010. Is there an ethical obligation to complete polio eradication? *Lancet* **375**:1340–1341. [8–11]

Faden, R., and S. Shebaya. 2010. Public health ethics. In: The Stanford Encyclopedia of Philosophy (summer 2010 edition). http://plato.stanford.edu/archives/sum2010/entries/publichealth-ethics/ (accessed 8 April 2011). [11]

Fahey, L., W. R. King, and V. K. Narayanan. 1981. Environmental scanning and forecasting in strategic planning: The state of the art. *Long Range Plann.* **14(1)**:32–39. [12, 14]

Farchy, D. J. 2005. A common good: Whither the global eradication of the measles virus? SSRN eLibrary. http://ssrn.com/paper=714302 (accessed 20 June 2010). [5]

Feilden, R., and O. F. Nielsen. 2001. Immunization and Health Reform: Making Reforms Work for Immunization. A Reference Guide. WHO/V&B/01.44. Geneva: WHO. [15]

Feinberg, J. 1984. The Moral Limits of the Criminal Law: Harm to Others. vol. 1. New York: Oxford Univ. Press. [8]

Fenner, F., A. J. Hall, and W. R. Dowdle. 1998. What is eradication? In: The Eradication of Infectious Diseases, ed. W. R. Dowdle and D. R. Hopkins, pp. 3–17. Dahlem Workshop Report, J. Lupp, series ed. Chichester: John Wiley & Sons. [1]

Fenner, F., D. A. Henderson, I. Arita, Z. Jezek, and I. D. Ladnyi. 1988. Smallpox and Its Eradication. Geneva: WHO. [2, 5, 9]

Ferroni, M., and A. Modi, eds. 2002. International Public Goods: Incentives, Measurement, and Financing. Amsterdam: Kluwer. [10]

Fine, P. E., and J. A. Clarkson. 1986. Individual versus public priorities in the determination of optimal vaccination policies. *Am. J. Epidemiol.* **124(6)**:1012–1020. [5]

Fine, P. E., and U. K. Griffiths. 2007. Global poliomyelitis eradication: Status and implications. *Lancet* **370**:132–133. [2]

Foege, W. H. 1971. Measles vaccination in Africa. In: Proc. of the Intl. Conf. on the Application of Vaccines against Viral, Rickettsial, and Bacterial Diseases of Man, pp. 207–212. Washington, D.C.: Pan American Health Organization. [3]

———. 1998. Thoughts on organization for disease eradication. In: The Eradication of Infectious Diseases, ed. W. R. Dowdle and D. R. Hopkins, pp. 187–191. Dahlem Workshop Reports, J. Lupp, series ed. Chichester: John Wiley & Sons. [7]

Frenk, J. 2006. Bridging the divide: Comprehensive reform to improve health in Mexico. WHO Commission on Social Determinants of Health, Nairobi, Kenya. http://www.who.int/social_determinants/resources/frenk.pdf (accessed 8 November 2010). [17]

Fulton, B. D., R. M. Scheffler, S. P. Sparkes, et al. 2011 Health workforce skill mix and task shifting in low income countries: A review of recent evidence. *Human Res. Health* **19(1)**:1. [19]

Gainotti, S., N. Moran, C. Petrini, and D. Shickle. 2008. Ethical models underpinning responses to threats to public health: A comparison of approaches to communicable disease control in Europe. *Bioethics* **22(9)**:466–476. [5]

Galindo, M. A., M. Santin, S. Resik, et al. 1998. The elimination of measles from Cuba. *Pan. Am. J. Public Health* **4**:171–177. [3]

Gambhir, M., M. Bockarie, D. Tisch, et al. 2010. Geographic and ecologic heterogeneity in elimination thresholds for the major vector-borne helminthic disease, lymphatic filariasis. *BMC Biology* **8(1)**:22. [6]

GAO. 2004. Emerging infectious diseases: Asian SARS outbreak challenged international and national responses. Report to the Chairman, Subcommittee on Asia and the Pacific, Committee on International Relations, House of Representatives. GAO-04-564. Washington, D.C.: GAO. [9]

Garrett, L. 2007. The challenge of global health. *Foreign Affairs* **86(1)**:14–38. [16]

Gauri, V., and P. Khaleghian. 2002. Immunization in developing countries: Its political and organizational determinants. *World Development* **30(12)**:2109–2132. [5]

GAVI Alliance. 2004. Guidelines for Preparing Proposals for GAVI/Vaccine Fund Investment (second draft, version 4). http://www.gavialliance.org/resources/13th_brd_Investment_case_guidelines_2.pdf (accessed 8 April 2011). [11]

———. 2006. Rotavirus and pneumococcal investment cases, notes from 29 November 2006 meeting, Doc A.1. http://www.gavialliance.org/resources/Rotavirus_Pneumo_Investment_Case_for_board_Nov06.pdf. (accessed 17 October 2010). [10]

———. 2010a. Approved support. http://www.gavialliance.org/performance/commitments/index.php (accessed 21 October 2010). [15]

———. 2010b. Goals. http://www.gavialliance.org/vision/strategy/goals/index.php (accessed 7 June 2010). [15]

————. 2010c. International finance facility for immunisation. http://www.iff-immunisation.org/ (accessed 17 October 2010). [10]

Geoffard, P. Y., and T. Philipson. 1997. Disease eradication private versus public vaccination. *Am. Econ. Rev.* **87(1)**:222–230. [9]

Gerencser, M., R. Van Lee, F. Napolitano, and C. Kelly. 2008. Megacommunities: How Leaders of Government, Business and Nonprofits Can Tackle Today's Global Challenges Together. New York: St. Martin's Press. [12]

Gersovitz, M., and J. S. Hammer. 2003. Infectious diseases, public policy, and the marriage of economics and epidemiology. *World Bank Research Observer* **18(2)**:129–157. [5]

GFATM. 2010. About the global fund. http://www.theglobalfund.org/en/about/?lang=en (accessed 25 May 2010). [15]

GIVS. 2011. Global immunization vision and strategy. http://www.who.int/immunization/givs/en/index.html (accessed 6 February 2011). [15]

Global Polio Eradication Initiative. 2010. Global Polio Eradication Initiative Strategic Plan 2010–2012. Geneva: WHO. [17]

Gold, M. R., J. E. Siegel, L. B. Russel, and M. C. Weinstein. 1996. Cost-effectiveness in Health and Medicine. New York: Oxford Univ. Press. [9]

Golding, M. 1972. Obligations to Future Generations. *The Monist* **56**:85. [8]

Goleman, D. 1995. Emotional Intelligence. New York: Bantam Books. [12]

————. 2000. Leadership that gets results. Product no. 4487. *Harvard Bus. Rev.* **78(3)**:1–13. [12]

Gonzalez, C. L. 1965. Mass Campaigns and General Health Services, Public Health papers, No. 29. Geneva: WHO. [15]

Goodman, R. A., K. L. Foster, F. L. Trowbridge, and J. P. Figueroa. 1998a. Global disease elimination and eradication as public health strategies. *Bull. WHO* **76(2)**:1–162. [2]

Goodman, R. A., D. R. Hopkins, I. Arita, et al. 1998b. When and how should eradication programs be implemented? In: The Eradication of Infectious Diseases, ed. W. R. Dowdle and D. R. Hopkins, pp. 193–205. Dahlem Workshop Reports, J. Lupp, series ed. Chichester: John Wiley & Sons. [7]

Grassly, N. C., C. Fraser, J. Wenger, et al. 2006. New strategies for the elimination of polio from India. *Science* **314**:1150–1153. [2]

Gravelle, H., and D. Smith. 2001. Discounting for health effects in cost-benefit and cost-effectiveness analysis. *Health Econ.* **10(7)**:587–599. [9]

Greenough, P. 1995. Intimidation, coercion and resistance in the final stages of the South Asian Smallpox Eradication Campaign, 1973–1975. *Soc. Sci. Med.* **41(5)**:633–645. [5]

Griffiths, U. K., P. Hanvoravongchai, V. Oliveira-Cruz, S. Mounier-Jack, and D. Balabanova. 2010. A toolkit for assessing the impacts of measles eradication activities on immunization services and health systems at country level: Developed for a multi-country study undertaken between July 2009–July 2010. http://www.cdprg.org/admin/editor_files/downloads/Measles_and_health_systems_toolkit.pdf (accessed 28 January 2011). [17]

Gupta, A. G., C. A. Moyera, and D. T. Stern. 2005. The economic impact of quarantine: SARS in Toronto as a case study. *J. Infect.* **50**:386–393. [9]

Gyapong, J., M. Gyapong, N. Yellu, et al. 2010. Integration of control of neglected tropical diseases into health-care systems: Challenges and opportunities. *Lancet* **375(9709)**:160–165. [4, 16, 19]

Gyapong, J., and N. A. Twum-Danso. 2006 Editorial: Global elimination of lymphatic filariasis: fact or fantasy? *Trop. Med. Intl. Health* **11(2)**:125–128. [19]

Haddad, D., C. Cross, B. Thylefors, et al. 2008. Health care at the end of the road: Opportunities from 20 years of partnership in onchocerciasis control. *Global Public Health* **3(2)**:187–196. [4]

Hall, B. F., and Anthony S. Fauci. 2009. Malaria control, elimination, and eradication: The role of the evolving biomedical research agenda. *J. Infect. Dis.* **200(11)**:1639–1643. [6]

Hart, H. L. A. 1994. The Concept of Law. Oxford: Clarendon Press. [8]

Hawkins, J. 2006. Justice and placebo controls. *Soc. Theory Prac.* **32(3)**:468. [8]

Hawkins, J., and E. J. Emanuel, eds. 2008. Exploitation and Developing Countries: The Ethics of Clinical Research. Princeton: Princeton Univ. Press. [8]

Hecht, R., and R. Shah. 2006. Recent trends and innovations in development assistance for health. In: Disease Control Priorities in Developing Countries (2nd edition), ed. D. T. Jamison et al. Washington, D.C.: World Bank. [19]

Henderson, D. A. 1987. Principles and lessons from the smallpox eradication programme. *Bull. WHO* **65**:535–46. [1]

———. 1998. Eradication: Lessons from the past. *Bull. WHO* **76(Suppl. 2)**:17–21. [6, 16]

Hinman, A. R. 1984. Prospects for disease eradication or elimination. *NY State J. Med.* **84(10)**:502–506. [1]

Hinman, A. R., and D. R. Hopkins. 1998. Lessons from previous eradication programs. In: The Eradication of Infectious Diseases, ed. W. R. Dowdle and D. R. Hopkins, pp. 19–31. Dahlem Workshop Report, J. Lupp, series ed. Chichester: John Wiley & Sons. [1, 5, 7]

Hissette, J. 1932. Mémoire on *Onchocerca volvulus* and ocular manifestations in the Belgian Congo. *Ann. Soc. Belge. Méd. Trop.* **12**:433–529. [4]

Homeida, M., E. Braide, E. Elhassan, et al. 2002. APOC's strategy of community-directed treatment with ivermectin (CDTI) and its potential for providing additional health services to the poorest populations. *Ann. Trop. Med. Parasitol.* **96(1)**:93–104. [4]

Hopkins, A. D. 2009. Challenges for the integration of mass drug administrations against multiple neglected tropical diseases. *Ann. Trop. Med. Parasitol.* **103(1)**:S23–S31. [4]

Hopkins, D. R. 2009. The allure of eradication. *Global Health Magazine*, http://www.globalhealthmagazine.com/top_stories/the_allure_of_eradication (accessed 11 October 2010). [1]

Horton, R. 2009. Venice statement: Global health initiatives and health systems. *Lancet* **374**:10–12. [15]

Howie, S. R. C., M. Antonio, A. Akisanya, et al. 2007. Re-emergence of *Haemophilus influenzae* type b (Hib) disease in The Gambia following successful elimination with conjugate Hib vaccine *Vaccine* **25(34)**:6305–6309. [6]

Hughes, J., and J. Weiss. 2007. Simple rules for making alliances work. *Harvard Bus. Rev.* **85(11)**:122–126. [12]

Hull, H. F. 2007. Pax polio. *Science* **275**:40–41. [2]

Hunt, T. 1937. Co-opetition. *Los Angeles Times*, Nov. 20, 1937, p. a4. [12]

Huppatz, C., C. Capuano, K. Palmer, P. Kelly, and D. Durrheim. 2009. Lessons from the Pacific programme to eliminate lymphatic filariasis: A case study of 5 countries. *BMC Infectious Diseases* **9(1)**:92. [6]

Hutubessy, R., D. Chisholm, T. Edejer, and WHO-CHOICE. 2003. Generalized cost-effectiveness analysis for national-level priority-setting in the health sector. *Cost Effect. Resource Allocation* **1(1)**:8. [9]

Ibarra, H., and J. Suesse. 1997. Building coalitions. Product no. 497055. *Harvard Bus. Rev.* **75(1)**:1–8. [12]

Igneski, V. 2006. Perfect and imperfect duties to aid. *Soc. Theory Prac.* **32(3)**:439–466. [8]

IHP+. International Health Partnership 2007. Available from http://www.internationalhealthpartnership.net/en/documents/category/official_ihp_documents. (accessed 1 December 2010). [16]

———. 2009. Taskforce on Innovative International Financing for Health Systems: More money for health, and more health for the money. www.internationalhealthpartnership.net//CMS_files/documents/taskforce_report_EN.pdf (accessed 1 December 2010). [16]

———. 2010. Welcome to the International Health Partnership and related initiatives. http://www.internationalhealthpartnership.net/en/home (accessed 7 June 2010). [15, 16]

IMF. 2010. IMF Survey Magazine interview: IMF moves on gold sales, SDR trading. 17 February 2010. http://www.imf.org/external/pubs/ft/survey/so/2010/int021710c.htm (accessed 16 October 2010). [10]

ITFDE. 2008. Updated table of diseases considered as candidates for global eradication by the International Task Force for disease eradication. http://www.cartercenter.org/resources/pdfs/news/health_publications/itfde/updated_disease_candidate_table.pdf (accessed 16 October 2010). [10]

ITI. 2010. Zithromax in the elimination of blinding trachoma: A program manager's guide. International Trachoma Initiative. http://www.trachoma.org/documents/ITIZithromaxManagersGuide_en_000.pdf (accessed 23 October 2010). [13]

Jamison, D. T., and J. S. Jamison. 2003. Discounting: Disease Control Priority Project Working Paper. Fogarty International Center: National Institute of Health [11].

Janis, I. L. 1982. Groupthink: Psychological Studies of Policy Decisions and Fiascoes, 2nd ed. New York: Houghton Mifflin. [12]

Jegede, A. S. 2007. What led to the Nigerian boycott of the polio vaccination campaign? *PLoS Med.* **4(3)**:e73. [16]

Jenner, W. 1801. The Origin of the Vaccine Inoculation. London: D. M. Shury. (Available at http://pyramid.spd.louisville.edu/~eri/fos/jenner_Origin.pdf, accessed 1 July 2010). [9]

Jonas, H. 1984. The Imperative of Responsibility: In Search of an Ethics for the Technological Age. Chicago: Univ. Chicago Press. [8]

Jones, G., R. W. Steketee, R. E. Black, Z. A. Bhutta, and S. S. Morris. 2003. Bellagio Child Survival Study Group. How many child deaths can we prevent this year? *Lancet* **362**:65–71. [15]

Kabatereine, N. B., M. N. Malecela, M. Lado, et al. 2010. How to (or not to) integrate vertical programmes for the control of major neglected tropical diseases in sub-Saharan Africa. *PLoS Negl. Trop. Dis.* **4(6)**:e755. [19]

Kabayo, J. P. 2002. Aiming to eliminate tsetse from Africa. *Trends Parasitol.* **18(11)**:473–475. [6]

Kant, I. 1785/1993. Grounding for the Metaphysics of Morals (trans. by J. W. Ellington). Indianapolis: Hackett Publ. [8]

Kanter, R. M. 1979. Power failure in management circuits. *Harvard Bus. Rev.* **57(7)**:65–76. [12]

Kates, J. 2010. Policy Brief, April 2010. The U.S. global health initiative: Key issues. http://www.kff.org/globalhealth/8063.cfm (accessed 2 July 2010). [15]

Kaufmann, J. R., and H. Feldbaum. 2009. Diplomacy and the polio immunization boycott in northern Nigeria. *Health Affairs* **28(4)**:1091. [2, 8, 10]

Keegan, R. A., A. Dabbagh, P. M. Strebel, and S. L. Cochi. 2011. Comparing measles with previous eradication programs: Enabling and constraining factors. *J. Infect. Dis.*, in press. [1]

Kelly, C., M. Gerencser, F. Napolitano, and R. Van Lee. 2007. The defining features of a megacommunity. *Strategy + Business* (June 12), http://www.strategy-business.com/article/li00029?pg=0 (accessed 2 February 2011). [14]

Kew, O. M., R. W. Sutter, E. M. de Gourville, W. R. Dowdle, and M. A. Pallansch. 2005. Vaccine-derived polioviruses and the endgame strategy for global polio eradication. *Annu. Rev. Microbiol.* **59**:587–635. [2]

Khan, M. M., and J. Ehreth. 2003. Costs and benefits of polio eradication: A long-run global perspective. *Vaccine* **21(7–8)**:702–705. [5]

Kirigia, J. M., and S. P. Barry. 2008. Health challenges in Africa and the way forward. *Intl. Arch. Med.* **18(1)**:27. [19]

Kotter, J. P. 2001. What leaders really do. *Harvard Bus. Rev.* **79(12)**:3–11. [12]

Kumar, A. 1990. Operational research need in guineaworm eradication programme. *J. Commun. Dis.* **22(4)**:236–242. [6]

Lahariya, C. 2007. Global eradication of polio: The case for "finishing the job." *Bull. WHO* **85(6)**:487–492. [5]

Lavery, J. V., P. O. Tinadana, T. W. Scott, et al. 2010. Towards a framework for community engagement in global health research. *Trends Parasitol.* **26**:279–283. [7]

Lawn, J. E., J. Rohde, S. Rifkin, et al. 2008. Alma-Ata: Rebirth and Revision 1. Alma-Ata 30 years on: Revolutionary, relevant, and time to revitalize. *Lancet* **372**:917–927. [15]

Lazcano-Ponce, E., B. Allen, and C. C. González. 2005. The contribution of international agencies to the control of communicable diseases. *Arch. Med. Res.* **36(6)**:731–738. [5]

Lee, J. W., B. Melgaard, H. F. Hull, D. Barakamfitiye, and J. M. Okwo-Bele. 1998. Ethical dilemmas in polio eradication. *Am. J. Public Health* **88**:130–132. [16]

Lemon, S. M., and S. E. Robertson. 1991. Global eradication of poliomyelitis: Recent progress, future prospects, and new research priorities. *Prog. Med. Virol.* **38**:42–45. [6]

Leyton-Brown, K., and Y. Shoham. 2008. Essentials of Game Theory: A Concise, Multidisciplinary Introduction. San Rafael, CA: Morgan & Claypool. [5]

Lockwood, D. N., and S. Suneetha. 2005. Leprosy: Too complex a disease for a simple elimination paradigm. *Bull. WHO* **83**:230–235. [6]

Loevinsohn, B., B. Aylward, R. Steinglass, et al. 2002. Impact of targeted programs on health systems: A case study of the polio eradication initiative. *Am. J. Public Health* **92(1)**:1923. [16, 17]

Lu, C., M. Schneider, P. Gubbins, et al. 2010. Public financing of health in developing countries: A cross-national systematic analysis. *Lancet* **375(9723)**:1375–1387. [16]

Malaria Elimination Group. 2011. http://www.malariaeliminationgroup.org/about (accessed 8 April 2011). [11]

Malaria Eradication Research Agenda. 2011. http://malera.tropika.net/ (accessed 8 April 2011). [11]

Malecela, M., W. Lazarus, U. Mwingira, et al. 2009. Eliminating LF: A Progress Report from Tanzania. *J. Lymphoedema* **4(1)**:10–12. [19]

Marais, B. J., and M. Pai. 2007. Recent advances in the diagnosis of childhood tuberculosis. *Arch. Dis. Child.* **92**:446–452. [6]

March, J. G., and H. A. Simon. 1958. Organizations. New York: John Wiley & Sons. [12]

Más Lago, P. 1999. Eradication of poliomyelitis in Cuba: A historical perspective. *Bull. WHO* **77(8)**:681–687. [9]

McCoy, D., S. Chand, and D. Sridhar. 2009. Global health funding: How much, where it comes from and where it goes. *Health Policy Plan.* **24(6)**:407–417. [16]

McCurry, J. 2008. G8 meeting disappoints on global health. *Lancet* **372(9634)**:191–194. [12]

McKinsey. 2010. The McKinsey 7 S framework. http://www.mindtools.com/pages/article/newSTR_91.htm (accessed 13 October 2010). [12]

Mectizan Donation Program. 2010. History. http://www.mectizan.org/history (accessed 25 May 2010). [15]

Melgaard, B., A. Creese, B. Aylward, et al. 1998. Disease eradication and health systems development. *Bull. WHO* **76(2)**:26–31. [1, 16, 17]

Merritt, M. 2007. Bioethics, philosophy, and global health. *Yale J. Health Policy, Law & Ethics* **7(2)**:273–317. [8]

Michael, E., M. N. Malecela, M. Zervos, and J. W. Kazura. 2008. Global eradication of lymphatic filariasis: the value of chronic disease control in parasite elimination programmes. *PLoS One* **13(3)**:e2936. [19]

Miles, S. A., and M. D. Watkins. 2007. The leadership team: Complementary strengths or conflicting agendas? *Harvard Bus. Rev.*, www.heidrick.com/PublicationsReports/Documents/HBR_LeadershipTeam.pdf (accessed 7 September 2010). [12]

Miller, M. A., S. Barrett, and D. A. Henderson. 2006. Control and eradication. In: Disease Control Priorities in Developing Countries, ed. D. Jamison et al., pp. 1163–1176. New York: World Bank and Oxford Univ. Press. [9]

Mills, A. 1983. Vertical vs horizontal health programmes in Africa: Idealism, pragmatism, resources and efficiency. *Soc. Sci. Med.* **17(24)**:1971–1981. [16, 17]

———. 2005. Mass campaigns versus general health services: What have we learnt in 40 years about vertical versus horizontal approaches? *Bull. WHO* **83(4)**:315–316. [15, 19]

Ministry of Health of Viet Nam. 2006. Multi-year plan for EPI: 2006–2010. http://www.gavialliance.org/resources/Vietnam_cMYP_2006_10.pdf (accessed 23 January 2010). [17]

MMWR. 1993. Recommendations of the International Task Force for Disease Eradication. *MMWR* **42(RR-16)**:1–38. [5]

Møgedal, S., and B. Stenson. 2000. Disease Eradication: Friend or Foe to the Health System? Synthesis report from field studies on the polio eradication initiative in Tanzania, Nepal and the Lao People's Democratic Republic. Geneva: WHO, Dept. of Vaccines and Biologicals. [16, 17]

Mohamed, A. J., P. Ndumbe, A. J. Hall, et al. 2009. Independent evaluation of major barriers to interrupting poliovirus transmission. Executive summary. http://www.polioeradication.org/content/general/Polio_Evaluation_CON.pdf (accessed 28 January 2011). [17]

Molyneux, D. H. 2009. 10 years of success in addressing lymphatic filariasiss. *Lancet* **373(9663)**:529–530. [19]

Molyneux, D. H., D. R. Hopkins, and N. Zagaria. 2004. Disease eradication, elimination and control: The need for accurate and consistent usage. *Trends Parasitol.* **20**:347–351. [6]

Moore, G. E. 1903. Principia Ethica. Cambridge: Cambridge Univ. Press. [8]

MPR News. 2009. Give MN: A look at the numbers http://minnesota.publicradio.org (accessed 7 September 2010). [12]

Narain, J. P., A. P. Dash, and B. Parnell. 2010. Elimination of neglected tropical diseases in the south-east Asia region of the World Health Organization. *Bull. WHO* **88**:206–210. [6]

Needham, C. A., and R. Canning. 2003. Global Disease Eradication: The Race for the Last Child. Washington, D.C.: ASM Press. [8]

Ngoumou, P., and J. F. Wash. 1993. A manuel for rapid epidemiological mapping of onchocerciasis. Document No. TDR/TDE/ONCHO/93.4. Geneva: WHO. [4]

NIAID and NIH. 2008a. NIAID malaria working group: NIAID research agenda for malaria. http://www.niaid.nih.gov/topics/malaria/documents/researchagenda.pdf (accessed 4 November 2010). [6]

———. 2008b. NIAID strategic plan for malaria research: Efforts to accelerate control and eradication of malaria through biomedical research. http://www.niaid.nih.gov/topics/malaria/documents/strategicplan.pdf (accessed 4 November 2010). [6]

Nohria, N., W. Joyce, and B. Roberson. 2003. What really works. *Harvard Bus. Rev.* **July**:42–52. [12]

Obadairo, C. 2010. Feasibility of measles eradication: stakeholder analysis. Global Technical Consultation Meeting on the Feasibility of Measles Eradication, July 28–30, 2010, at Washington, D.C., Washington, D.C.: PAHO. [2]

Obadare, E. 2005. A crisis of trust: History, politics, religion and the polio controversy in northern Nigeria. *Patt. Prejudice* **39(3)**:265. [10, 16]

OECD. 1998. Effects of European Union accession, Part 1: Budgeting and financial control, SIGMA Paper No. 19, Appendix 3: List of Useful Terms. http://ideas.repec.org/p/oec/govaac/19-en.html (accessed 17 October 2010). [12]

———. 2005. Paris Declaration on aid effectiveness. http://www.oecd.org/dataoecd/11/41/34428351.pdf (accessed 17 October 2010). [12, 16]

———. 2008a. The Paris Declaration and Accra Agenda for Action: Full related documentation. http://www.oecd.org/dataoecd/11/41/34428351.pdf (accessed 25 May 2010). [15]

———. 2008b. Survey on monitoring the Paris Declaration: Making aid more effective by 2010. http://www.oecd.org/document/0/0,3343, en_2649_3236398_41203264_1_1_1_1,00.html (accessed 22 November 2010). [16]

Oliveira-Cruz, V., C. Kurowski, and A. Mills. 2003. Delivery of priority health services: Searching for synergies within the vertical versus horizontal debate. *J. Intl. Develop.* **15**:67–86. [15]

Oliveira Cruz, V., and B. McPake. 2010. The "aid contract" and its compensation scheme: A case study of the performance of the Ugandan health sector. *Soc. Sci. Med.* **71(7)**:1357–1365. [19]

O'Neil, J. 1875. On the presence of filaria in craw-craw. *Lancet* **1**:265–266. [4]

O'Neill, O. 2002. Autonomy and Trust in Bioethics. Cambridge: Cambridge Univ. Press. [8]

———. 2005. The dark side of human rights. *Intl. Affairs* **81**:427–439. [8]

Oomman, N., M. Bernstein, and S. Rosenzweig. 2007. Following the Funding for HIV/AIDS: A Comparative Analysis of the Funding Practices of PEPFAR, the Global Fund and World Bank MAP in Mozambique, Uganda and Zambia. Washington, D.C.: Center for Global Development. [12]

Ooms, G., K. Decoster, K. Miti, et al. 2010. Crowding out: Are relations between international health aid and government health funding too complex to be captured in averages only? *Lancet* **375(9723)**:1403–1405. [16]

Ottesen, E. A., W. R. Dowdle, F. Fenner, et al. 1998. How is eradication to be defined and what are the biological criteria? In: The Eradication of Infectious Diseases, ed. W. R. Dowdle and D. R. Hopkins, pp. 47–59. Dahlem Workshop Report, J. Lupp, series ed. Chichester: John Wiley & Sons. [1, 5, 7]

Ottesen, E. A., P. J. Hooper, M. Bradley, and G. Biswas. 2008. The global programme to eliminate lymphatic filariasis: Health impact after 8 years. *PLoS Negl. Trop. Dis.* **2(10)**:e317. [6, 13]

Oxfam. 2002. False hope or new start? The global fund to fight HIV/AIDS, TB, and Malaria. http://www.oxfam.org.uk/resources/policy/health/downloads/bp24_globalfund.pdf (accessed 8 April 2011). [16]

PAHO. 2003. 44th Direction Council. Resolution CD44.R1. Sustaining immunization programs: Elimination of rubella and congenital rubella syndrome. http://www.paho.org/English/gov/cd/cd44-r1-e.pdf (accessed 27 January 2011). [3]

————. 2004. XVI Meeting: Final report of the technical advisory group on vaccine-preventable diseases, Mexico City, Nov. 3–5, pp. 1–55. http://www.paho.org/English/AD/FCH/IM/TAG16_2004_FinalReport_Eng.pdf (accessed 27 January 2011). [3]

Panda, A., and R. K. Gupta. 2001. Understanding organizational culture: A perspective on roles for leaders. *Vikalpa* **26(4)**:1–19. [12]

Parsonage, M., and H. Neuburger. 1992. Discounting and health benefits. *Health Econ.* **1(1)**:71–76. [9]

Patel, P., B. Roberts, L. Conteh, S. Guy, and L. Lee-Jones. 2010. A review of global mechanisms for tracking official development assistance for health in countries affected by armed conflict. *Health Policy*, doi:10.1016/j.healthpol.2010.08.007. [19]

PATH's Rotavirus Vaccine Program. 2006. Accelerating the Introduction of Rotavirus Vaccines into GAVI-Eligible Countries. http://www.gavialliance.org/resources/Rotavirus_Investment_Case_Oct06.pdf (accessed 8 April 2011). [11]

Paul, Y. 2005. Polio eradication programme: Some ethical issues. *Indian J. Med. Ethics* **2(4)**:115. [8]

Paul, Y., and A. Dawson. 2005. Some ethical issues arising from polio eradication programmes in India. *Bioethics* **19(4)**:393. [8]

Pearson, M., B. Kent, and P. Sok. 2008. Global health partnerships: Deploying vertical financing to support horizontal efforts. DFID Health Resource Centre. http://network.human-scale.net/docs/DOC-1257 (accessed 27 January 2011). [16]

Perera, M., M. Whitehead, and D. H. Molyneaux. 2007. Neglected patients with a neglected disease? A qualitative study of lymphatic filariasis. *PLoS Negl. Trop. Dis.* **1**:e128. [6]

Piva, P., and R. Dodd. 2009. Where did all the aid go? An in-depth analysis of increased health aid flows over the past 10 years. *Bull. WHO* **87(12)**:930–939. [19]

Polio Eradication Initiative. 2010a. Financial resource requirements. http://www.polioeradication.org/fundingbackground.asp (accessed 25 May 2010). [15]

————. 2010b. Strategic plan 2010–2012. http://www.polioeradication.org/Portals/0/Document/StrategicPlan/StratPlan2010_2012_ENG.pdf (accessed 6 February 2011). [15]

Pope, C., and N. Mays, eds. 1996. Qualitative Research in Health Care. London: BMJ Publishing Group. [17]

Powers, M., and R. Faden. 2006. Social Justice: the Moral Foundations of Public Health and Health Policy. Oxford: Oxford Univ. Press. [11]

Rajaratnam, J. K., J. R. Marcus, A. D. Flaxman, et al. 2010. Neonatal, postneonatal, childhood, and under-5 mortality for 187 countries, 1970–2010: A systematic analysis of progress towards Millenium Development Goal 4. *Lancet* **375**:1988–2008. [15]

Ravishankar, N., P. Gubbins, R. J. Cooley, et al. 2009. Financing of global health: Tracking development assistance for health from 1990 to 2007. *Lancet* **373**:2113–2124. [15, 17]

Renne, E. 2006. Perspectives on polio and immunization in Northern Nigeria. *Soc. Sci. Med.* **63**:1857–1869. [16, 18]

Ridley, H. 1945. Ocular Onchocerciasis, including an investigation in the Gold Coast. *Br. J. Ophthalmol.* **10(Suppl)**:1–58. [4]

Rifkin, S. B., and G. Walt. 1986. Why health improves: Defining the issues concerning comprehensive primary health care and selective primary health care. *Soc. Sci. Med.* **23(6)**:559–566. [17]

Ritchie, J., and L. Spencer. 1994. Qualitative data analysis for applied policy research. In: Analyzing Qualitative Data, ed. B. A. Burgess, pp. 173–194. London: Routledge. [17]

Robels, R. 1917. Enfermedad nueva in Guatemala. *Juventud Med.* **17**:97–115. [4]

Roberts, J. 2004. Alliances, Coalitions and Partnerships. Gabriola Island, BC: New Society Publ. [12]

Roberts, J., E. Neumann, C. W. Guckel, and R. B. Highton. 1986. Onchocerciasis in Kenya 9, 11, and 18 years after elimination of the vector. *Bull. WHO* **64**:667–681. [4]

Rockefeller Foundation. 2003. Human resources: A joint learning initiative. http://www.rockefellerfoundation.org/uploads/files/ad7cea0d-33f9-4de3-82c1-dabd88f5ca4f-03hrh.pdf (accessed 23 November 2010). [16]

Rogers, D. J., and S. E. Randolph. 2002. A response to the aim of eradicating tsetse from Africa. *Trends Parasitol.* **18**:534–536. [6]

Rogers, E. M. 2003. Diffusion of Innovations, 5th edition. New York: Free Press. [18]

Ropero-Alvarez, A. M., H. J. Kurtis, M. C. Danovaro-Holliday, C. Ruiz Matus, and J. K. Andrus. 2009. Expansion of seasonal influenza vaccination in the Americas. *BMC Public Health* **9**:361. [3]

Rosenstein, S., and L. Garrett. 2006. Olio's Return, a WHO-Done it? *The American Interest* **1(3)**:19–27. [16]

Rowden, R. 2010. Why health advocates must get involved in development economics: The case of the International Monetary Fund. *Intl. J. Health Serv.* **40(1)**:183–187. [19]

Ryman, T. K., V. Dietz, and K. L. Cairns. 2008. Too little but not too late: Results of a literature review to improve routine immunization programs in developing countries. *BMC Health Serv. Res.* **8**:134. [5]

Salisbury, D. 1998. Report of the workgroup on disease elimination/eradication and sustainable health development. *Bull. WHO* **76(2)**:72–79. [17]

Samba, E. M. 1994. The Onchocerciasis Control Program in West Africa: An Example of Effective Public Health Management. Geneva: WHO. [4]

Sangrujee, N., R. J. Duintjer Tebbens, V. M. Cáceres, and K. M. Thompson. 2003. Policy decision options during the first 5 years following certification of polio eradication. *Medscape Gen. Med.* **5(4)**:35. [9]

Sathyamala, C., M. Onkar, R. Dasgupta, and R. Priya. 2005. Polio eradication initiative in India: Deconstructing the GPEI. *Intl. J. Health Serv.* **35(2)**:361–383. [16]

Sauerbrey, M. 2008. The onchocerciasis elimination program for the Americas. *Ann. Trop. Med. Parasitol.* **102(1)**:S25–S29. [4]

Schieber, G., C. Baeza, D. Kress, and M. Maier. 2006. Financing health systems in the 21st century. In: Disease Control Priorities in Developing Countries (2nd edition), ed. D. T. Jamison et al. Washington, D.C.: World Bank. [19]

Schmunis, G. A., F. Zicker, and A. Moncayo. 1996. Interruption of Chagas' disease transmission through vector elimination. *Lancet* **348**:1171. [6]

Schwarz, E. C., J. Renk, A. D. Hopkins, R. Huss, and A. Foster. 1999. A method to determine the coverage of ivermectin distribution programs in onchocerciasis control *Ann. Trop. Med. Parasitol.* **92(7)**:793–796. [4]

Shiffman, J. 2006. Donor funding priorities for communicable disease control in the developing world. *Health Policy Plan.* **21(6)**:411–420. [5]

Shigayeva, A., R. Atun, M. McKee, and R. Coker. 2010. Health systems, communicable diseases and integration. *Health Policy Plan.* **25(Suppl. 1)**:i4–i20. [17]

Shulman, S. T. 2004. The history of pediatric infectious diseases. *Pediatric Res.* **55**:163–176. [9]

Singer, P. 1997. The drowning child and the expanding circle. *New Internationalist*, http://www.newint.org/features/1997/04/05/drowning/ (accessed 8 April 2011). [8]

Sinha, K. 2008. Study finds polio drive counter-productive. *The Times of India*, http://timesofindia.indiatimes.com/Study_finds_polio_drive_counter-productive/rssarticleshow/3089610.cms (accessed 1 June 2008). [16]

Slonim, D., E. Svandova, P. Strand, and C. Benes. 1995. History of poliomyelitis in the Czech Republic. Part III. *Cen. Europ. J. Public Health* **3(3)**:124–126. [9]

Smith, C. E. 1964. Factors in the transmission of virus infections from animals to man. *Sci. Basis Med. Annu. Rev.*:125–150. [5]

Smith, R. D., R. Beaglehole, D. Woodward, and N. Drager, eds. 2003. Global Public Goods for Health: Health Economic and Public Health Perspectives. Oxford: Oxford Univ. Press. [8]

Smith, R. D., D. Woodward, A. Acharya, R. Beaglehole, and N. Drager. 2004. Communicable disease control: A "Global Public Good" perspective. *Health Policy Plan.* **19(5)**:271–278. [5]

Surber, J. P. 1977. Obligations to future generations: Explorations and problemata. *J. Value Inquiry* **11(2)**:107. [8]

Sutter, R. W., and S. L. Cochi. 1997. Comment: Ethical dilemmas in worldwide polio eradication programs. *Am. J. Public Health* **87(6)**:913–915. [8]

Sutter, R. W., T. J. John, H. Jain, et al. 2010. Immunogenicity of bivalent types 1 and 3 oral poliovirus vaccine: A randomised, double-blind, controlled trial. *Lancet* **376**:1682–1688. [2]

Tambini, G., J. K. Andrus, J. W. Fitzsimmons, and M. R. Periago. 2006. Regional immunization programs as a model for strengthening cooperation among nations. *Pan. Am. J. Public Health* **20(1)**:54–59. [3, 9]

Tangcharoensathien, V., and W. Patcharanarumol. 2010. Global health initiatives: Opportunities or challenges? *Health Policy Plan.* **25**:101–103. [15]

Tangermann, R. H., H. F. Hull, B. Nkowane, H. Everts, and R. B. Aylward. 2000. Eradication of poliomyelitis in countries affected by conflict. *Bull. WHO* **78**:330–338. [2]

Taylor, C., H. Cordeiro, and F. Cutts. 1995. Taylor Commission. The Impact of the Expanded Program on Immunization and the Polio Eradication Initiative on Health Systems in the Americas. Washington, D.C.: PAHO. [16, 17]

Taylor, C., F. Cutts, and M. Taylor. 1997. Ethical dilemmas in current planning for polio eradication. *Am. J. Public Health* **87(6)**:922–925. [16, 17]

Taylor, C., and R. J. Waldman. 1998. Designing eradication programs to strengthen primary health care. In: The Eradication of Infectious Diseases, ed. W. R. Dowdle and D. R. Hopkins, pp. 145–155. Dahlem Workshop Report, J. Lupp, series ed. Chichester: John Wiley & Sons. [1, 17]

Taylor, S. 2009. Political epidemiology: Strengthening socio-political analysis for mass immunisation-lessons from the smallpox and polio programmes. *Global Public Health* **4(6)**:546–560. [5, 18]

Thompson, K. M., and R. J. Duintjer Tebbens. 2006. Retrospective cost-effectiveness analyses for polio vaccination in the United States. *Risk Analysis* **26(6)**:1423–1440. [9]

———. 2007. Eradication versus control for poliomyelitis: An economic analysis. *Lancet* **369(9570)**:1363–1371. [1, 5, 8–10]

———. 2008a. The case for cooperation in managing and maintaining the end of poliomyelitis: Stockpile needs and coordinated OPV cessation. *Medscape J. Med.* **10(8)**:190. [5]

———. 2008b. Using system dynamics to develop policies that matter: Global management of poliomyelitis and beyond. *System Dynamics Rev.* **24(4)**:433–449. [9, 10]

Thompson, K. M., R. J. Duintjer Tebbens, and M. A. Pallansch. 2006. Evaluation of response scenarios to potential polio outbreaks using mathematical models. *Risk Analysis* **26(6)**:1541–1556. [9]

Thompson, K. M., R. J. Duintjer Tebbens, M. A. Pallansch, et al. 2008. The risks, costs, and benefits of global policies for managing polio after eradication. *Am. J. Public Health* **98(7)**:1322–30. [9]

Thylfors, B., M. M. Alleman, and N. Twum-Danso. 2008. Operational lessons from 20 years of the Mectizan donation program for the control of onchocerciasis. *Trop. Med. Intl. Health* **13(5)**:689–696. [13]

Tomori, O., C. Maher, S. Essien, et al. 2010. 19th Meeting of the expert review committee on polio eradication and routine immunization in Nigeria, 22–24 March 2010, Minna, Nigeria. http://www.comminit.com/files/FinalReport-19thERCMeeting.pdf (accessed 13 March 2011). [18]

Travis, P., S. Bennett, A. Haines, et al. 2004. Overcoming health-systems constraints to achieve the Millennium Development Goals. *Lancet* **364(9437)**:900–906. [17]

Ulmer, J. B., and M. A. Liu. 2002. Science and society—vaccines: Ethical issues for vaccines and immunization. *Nat. Rev. Immun.* **2**:291. [8]

UN. 1948. The Universal Declaration of Human Rights, Article 25. http://www.un.org/en/documents/udhr/index.shtml (accessed 12 February 2011). [8]

———. 1966. International Covenant of Economic, Social and Cultural Rights (ICESCR), Article 12. http://www2.ohchr.org/english/law/cescr.htm (accessed 12 February 2011). [8]

Unger, J.-P., P. De Paepe, and A. Green. 2003. A code of best practice for disease control programs to avoid damaging health care services in developing countries. *Intl. J. Health Plan. Manag.* **18**:S27–S39. [16]

UNICEF. 2010. Knowledge, Attitudes and Practices (KAP) on Polio "Plus" in the 107 High Risk Blocks of UP and Bihar, in press. [18]

UNICEF, UNDP, World Bank, and WHO. 2008. Community-directed Interventions for Major Health Problems in Africa: A Multi-country Study. Special Program for Research and Training in Tropical Diseases. Geneva: WHO. [16, 17]

UNPD. 2009. World population prospects: The 2008 revision population database. http://esa.un.org/UNPP/ (accessed 27 January 2011). [17]

U.S. FDA. 2009. What is a serious adverse event? *MedWatch The FDA Safety Information and Adverse Event Reporting Program*, http://www.fda.gov/Safety/MedWatch/HowToReport/ucm053087.htm (accessed 3 November 2010). [13]

U.S. Global Health Initiative. 2010. U.S. Global Health Initiative: Key Issues—Kaiser Family Foundation Policy Brief. http://www.kff.org/globalhealth/8063.cfm (accessed 23 November 2010). [16]

van Hout, B. A. 1998. Discounting costs and effects: A reconsideration. *Health Econ.* **7(7)**:581–594. [9]

Vashishtha, V. M. 2009. Why tuberculosis is a difficult disease to target for control or elimination? *Indian J. Pediatr.* **46**:82–83. [6]

Vashishtha, V. M., T. J. John, R. K. Agarwal, and A. Kalra. 2008. Universal immunization program and polio eradication in India. *Indian J. Pediatr.* **45(10)**:807–813. [16]

Verwieji, M., and A. Dawson. 2004. Ethical principles for collective immunization programmes. *Vaccine* **22**:3122–3126. [8]

Vujicic, M. 2010. Scaling up the health workforce in the public sector: the role of government fiscal policy. *World Hosp. Health Serv.* **46(3)**:20–23. [19]

Wakabi, W. 2009. Africa sees obstacles to guinea worm disease eradication. *Lancet* **373(9670)**:1159. [17]

Wallace, A. 2005. Getting 1 + 1 to equal three: Best practices for maximizing benefits and overcoming barriers to the integration of lymphatic filariasis elimination with other health interventions in Tanzania. Unpublished masters thesis, Rollins School of Public Health, Global Health Department, Emory University, Atlanta. [15]

Wallace, A., V. Dietz, and K. L. Cairns. 2009. Integration of immunization services with other health interventions in the developing world: What works and why? Systematic literature review. *Trop. Med. Intl. Health* **14(1–9)**. [15]

Walsh, J. A., and K. S. Warren. 1979. Selective primary health care. *N. Engl. J. Med.* **301(18)**:967–974. [17]

———. 1980. Selective primary health care: An interim strategy for disease control in developing countries. *Soc. Sci. Med.* **14(2)**:145–163. [16]

Wassilak, S., and W. Orenstein. 2010. Challenges faced by the global polio eradication initiative. *Expert Rev. Vaccines* **9(5)**:447–449. [17]

Weil, D. E. C. 2000. Advancing tuberculosis control within reforming health systems. *Intl. J. Tuberc. Lung Dis.* **4**:597–605. [15]

WHO. 1946. Constitution. http://www.who.int/governance/eb/constitution/en/index.html (accessed 12 February 2011). [8]

———. 1978. Primary health care: Report on the international conference on primary health care, Alma-Ata, USSR. http://whqlibdoc.who.int/publications/9241800011.pdf (accessed 23 November 2010). [16]

———. 1988. Global eradication of poliomyelitis by the year 2000. World Health Assembly Resolution 41.28. Geneva: WHO. [2, 16]

———. 1998. Global disease elimination and eradication as public health strategies. *Bull. WHO* **76(2)**:1–162. [1]

————. 2000a. Preparing and implementing a national plan to eliminate lymphatic filariasis: A guideline for programme managers. http://www.filariasis.org/pdfs/Press%20Centre/Training%20Material/pmginco.pdf (accessed 23 October 2010). [13]

————. 2000b. The world health report 2000. Health systems: Improving performance. http://www.who.int/whr/2000/en/ (accessed 27 January 2011). [16]

————. 2001a. Checklist and indicators for optimizing the impact of polio activities on EPI. http://www.polioeradication.org/content/publications/checklist_optimizeactivities.pdf (accessed 23 November 2010). [16]

————. 2001b. Macroeconomics and health: Investing in health for economic development. Report of the Commission on Macroeconomics and Health. http://www.paho.org/English/HDP/HDD/Sachs.pdf (accessed 1 July 2010). [9]

————. 2001c. Transmission of wild poliovirus type 2: Apparent global interruption. *W. Epidem. Rec.* **76**:95–97. [9]

————. 2002. Understanding barriers to polio eradication in Uttar Pradesh: Final report. http://www.comminit.com/en/node/220372/303 (accessed 23 November 2010). [16]

————. 2003a. Global Polio Eradication Initiative: Estimated external financial resource requirements 2004–2008. Geneva: WHO. [2]

————. 2003b. SARS outbreak contained worldwide: Threat remains and more research needed, says WHO. http://www.who.int/mediacentre/news/releases/2003/pr56/en/ (accessed 1 July 2010). [9]

————. 2004. High-level forum on the health MDGs. www.who.int/hdp/en/summary.pdf (accessed 23 November 2010). [16]

————. 2006a. Action against worms. Issue 6. http://www.who.int/wormcontrol/newsletter/PPC6_Eng.pdf (accessed 23 October 2010). [13]

————. 2006b. Opportunities for global health initiatives in the health systems action agenda, working paper 4. http://www.who.int/management/Making%20HSWork%204.pdf (accessed 27 January 2011). [16]

————. 2006c. Preventive chemotherapy in human helminthiasis. http://whqlibdoc.who.int/publications/2006/9241547103_eng.pdf (accessed 21 February 2011). [4, 13]

————. 2006d. Trachoma control: A guide for programme managers. http://whqlibdoc.who.int/publications/2006/9241546905_eng.pdf (accessed 23 October 2010). [13]

————. 2006e. The world health report 2006: Working together for health. http://www.who.int/whr/2006/en/ (accessed 23 November 2010). [16]

————. 2007a. Everybody's business: Strengthening health systems to improve health outcomes. WHO's Framework for Action. Geneva: WHO. [15–17]

————. 2007b. Health of migrants: Report by the Secretariat, 20 December 2007. EB122/11. http://apps.who.int/gb/ebwha/pdf_files/EB122/B122_11-en.pdf (accessed 6 December 2010). [18]

————. 2007c. Spending on health: A global overview. http://www.who.int/mediacentre/factsheets/fs319/en/print.html (accessed 1 July 2010). [9]

————. 2008a. Guide for standardization of economic evaluations of immunization programmes, WHO/IVB/08.14. http://whqlibdoc.who.int/hq/2008/WHO_IVB_08.14_eng.pdf (accessed 1 July 2010). [9–11]

————. 2008b. Thematic evaluation of poliomyelitis eradication. Executive Board of the World Health Assembly. Geneva: WHO. [2]

————. 2008c. The World Health Report 2008. Primary health care, now more than ever. www.who.int/whr/2008/en/ (accessed 23 November 2010). [16]

————. 2009. Measles vaccines: WHO position paper. *W. Epidem. Rec.* **35(89)**:349–360. [3]

————. 2010a. Global eradication of measles: Report of the Secretariat, WHO/A63/18. http://apps.who.int/gb/ebwha/pdf_files/WHA63/A63_18-en.pdf (accessed 1 July 2010). [11, 16, 17]

————. 2010b. Global immunization vision and strategy. http://www.who.int/immunization/givs/en/ (accessed 7 June 2010). [15]

————. 2010c. Global Polio Eradication Initiative: Strategic Plan 2010–2012. WHO Document WHO/Polio/10.01. Geneva: WHO. [2]

————. 2010d. Monitoring drug coverage for preventive chemotherapy. http://whqlibdoc.who.int/publications/2010/9789241599993_eng.pdf (accessed 21 February 2011). [4]

————. 2010e. Monitoring progress towards measles elimination. *W. Epidem. Rec.* **85**:490–495. [1]

————. 2010f. Outbreaks following importations of wild poliovirus into countries of the WHO African, European and South-East Asian Regions: January 2009–September 2010. *W. Epidem. Rec.* **85**:445–452. [2, 16]

————. 2011. WHO African region: Nigeria. Expanded programme on immunization. http://www.who.int/countries/nga/areas/epi/en/index.html (accessed 2 January 2011). [18]

WHO/APOC. 2007a. Revitalising health care delivery in sub-Saharan Africa: The potential of community-directed treatment to strengthen health systems. http://www.who.int/apoc/publications/EN_HealthCare07_7_3_08.pdf (accessed 17 February 2011). [4]

————. 2007b. Year 2007 progress report of WHO/APOC. http://www.who.int/apoc/publications/progress_report_jaf13_2007_en.pdf (accessed 18 February 2011). [4]

————. 2009 Informal consultation on elimination of onchocerciasis transmission using current tools in Africa "Shrinking the Map." Ouagadougou, Burkina Faso, February 25–27, 2009 [4]

WHO Maximizing Positive Synergies Collaborative Group. 2009. An assessment of interactions between global health initiatives and country health systems. *Lancet* **373**:2137–2169. [1, 15, 16]

WHO Regional Office for Africa. 2007. In-depth evaluation of the reaching every district approach in the African region. http://www.who.int/immunization/sage/1_AFRO_1_RED_Evaluation_Report_2007_Final.pdf (accessed 8 November, 2010). [17]

————. 2010. Integration of child survival interventions with immunization services. http://www.afro.who.int/index.php?Itemid=2572 (accessed 1 August 2010). [17]

WHO Strategic Advisory Group of Experts. 2010. Impact of new vaccines introduction on immunization and health systems. Report of an ad-hoc working group. http://www.who.int/immunization/sage/NUVI_IS_HS_final_Refs_12_April_2010.pdf (accessed 21 October 2010). [15]

WHO/TDR. 2008. Community-directed interventions for major health problems in Africa: A multi-country study. Final report 2008. http://apps.who.int/tdr/publications/tdr-research-publications/community-directed-interventions-health-problems/pdf/cdi_report_08.pdf (accessed 1 March 2011). [4, 19]

WHO, UNICEF, and World Bank. 2009. State of the World's Vaccines and Immunization, 3rd ed. Geneva: World Health Organization. [9]

WHO, UNICEF., and USAID. 2000. Communication for routine immunization and polio eradication: A synopsis of five sub-Saharan country case studies. http://indexmedicus.afro.who.int/iah/fulltext/synopsis-fivesubsaharan.pdf (accessed 27 January 2011). [18]

Williams, G. A., and R. B. Miller. 2002. Change the way you persuade. *Harvard Bus. Rev.* **May**:65–73. [12]

Windsor, D. A. 1998. Equal rights for parasites. *Bioscience* **48(4)**:244. [8]

Woodward, D., and R. D. Smith. 2003. The global public goods for health concept. In: Global Public Goods for Health, ed. R. D. Smith et al. Oxford: Oxford Univ. Press. [8]

World Bank. 1993. World Bank Development Report 1993: Investing in Health. New York: Oxford Univ. Press. [3]

———. 2007. Healthy development: The World Bank strategy for HNP results. http://siteresources.worldbank.org/HEALTHNUTRITIONANDPOPULATION/Resources/281627-1154048816360/HNPStrategyFINALApril302007.pdf (accessed 23 November 2010). [16]

———. 2011a. Global partnership to eliminate riverblindness. http://go.worldbank.org/F5NNFM6K40 (accessed 19 February 2011). [4]

———. 2011b. GNI per capita, Atlas method (current US$). http://data.worldbank.org/indicator/NY.GNP.PCAP.CD (accessed 22 Jan 2010). [17]

World Bank/APOC. 2010. Press Release No: 2011/239/AFR ABUJA, December 10, 2010. http://web.worldbank.org/WBSITE/EXTERNAL/COUNTRIES/AFRICAEXT/0,,contentMDK:22788056~menuPK:2246551~pagePK:2865106~piPK:2865128~theSitePK:258644,00.html (accessed 17 February 2010). [4]

World Economic Forum. 2009. Managing our future water needs. www.weforum.org/pdf/water/WaterInitiativeGlance.pdf (accessed 27 January 2011). [12]

World Health Assembly. 1988. Global Eradication of Poliomyelitis by the Year 2000, Resolution 41.28. Geneva: WHO. [5, 9]

Yahya, M. 2006. Polio vaccines – difficult to swallow: The story of a controversy in northern Nigeria. http://www.eldis.org/vfile/upload/1/document/0708/DOC21227.pdf (accessed 27 January 2011). [16]

Zimmerman, P. A., C. R. Katholi, M. C. Wooten, N. Lang-Unnasch, and T. R. Unnasch. 1994. Recent evolutionary history of American *Onchocerca volvulus*, based on analysis of a tandemly repeated DNA sequence family. *Mol. Biol. Evol.* **11(3)**:384–392. [4]

Subject Index